Coping with Caring

Coping with Caring
A Nurse's Guide to Better Health and Job Satisfaction

Meredith Mealer

Photos By: Rowan Waldman

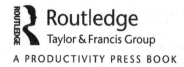

Routledge
Taylor & Francis Group

A PRODUCTIVITY PRESS BOOK

First edition published in 2020
by Routledge/Productivity Press
52 Vanderbilt Avenue, 11th Floor New York, NY 10017
2 Park Square, Milton Park, Abingdon, Oxon OX14 4RN, UK

International Standard Book Number-13: 978-1-138-32824-2 (Paperback)
International Standard Book Number-13: 978-1-138-33893-7 (Hardback)
International Standard Book Number-13: 978-0-429-44877-5 (eBook)

Library of Congress Cataloging-in-Publication Data

Names: Mealer, Meredith, author.
Title: Coping with caring : a nurse's guide to better health and job
satisfaction / Meredith Mealer.
Description: Boca Raton : Taylor & Francis, 2020. | "A Routledge title, part
of the Taylor & Francis imprint, a member of the Taylor & Francis Group,
the academic division of T&F Informa plc." | Includes bibliographical
references and index.
Identifiers: LCCN 2019013310 (print) | LCCN 2019014195 (ebook) |
ISBN 9780429448775 (e-Book) | ISBN 9781138328242 (pbk. : alk. paper) |
ISBN 9781138338937 (hardback : alk. paper)
Subjects: LCSH: Nursing—Psychological aspects. | Job stress—Prevention.
Classification: LCC RT86 (ebook) | LCC RT86 .M42 2020 (print) | DDC
610.73—dc23
LC record available at https://lccn.loc.gov/2019013310

Visit the Taylor & Francis Web site at
http://www.taylorandfrancis.com

Contents

Preface: Coping with Caring

My passion for wellness and behavioral interventions to build resilience in nurses and other healthcare clinicians began over 15 years ago, when I left bedside nursing in the intensive care unit (ICU) and started my career as a researcher in critical care. I was involved in a clinical research study that was exploring quality of life outcomes in patients who were survivors of their critical illness. There were several quality of life surveys that our research team would administer to these patients, but one in particular caught my attention, which was a short inventory of stress and symptoms of posttraumatic stress disorder (PTSD).

The survey is called the Posttraumatic Symptom Scale (PTSS-10) and includes 10 questions addressing the diagnostic symptoms clusters of PTSD, which include intrusion, avoidance, and hypervigilance. The PTSS-10 was based on the model of stress and the interaction between the environment, the individual, and the stress reaction. As I was reading through the questions and administering the survey to study participants, I started to reflect upon my experiences as a bedside nurse in the ICU. My job was pretty stressful, and I did recall having issues with sleep, anxiety, feeling guilty, or regret about not being able to save a particular patient; on occasion, I would sometimes fear taking care of a patient that would remind me of a similar patient that I had cared for where the outcome was not favorable.

Anecdotally, I started questioning former colleagues when they left the bedside with "do you remember all the good times we had working in the unit together" and "why did you leave?" All of the stories were contextually unique, but the themes were all quite similar and included anxiety, sleep problems, nightmares, fear, guilt, and regret.

I worked in a hospital where there wasn't a critical response team; instead, each of the ICUs was assigned to areas of the hospital, and in the event of a cardiopulmonary arrest, an ICU nurse would have to respond and run the code along with the critical care physician. The unit assignments were usually close in proximity, but sometimes, if responding to radiology or the MRI scanner, the nurse would have to travel quite a distance to get to the patient. The hospital overhead pager would go off, and the operator would announce "Code Blue, medical unit, room 7101...Code Blue, medical unit, room 7101...Code Blue, medical unit, room 7101," and the ICU nurse would have to drop everything they were doing and run to the location. Some nurses enjoyed being the code responder, and some preferred not to be the responder, but all of the nurses in the unit would eventually be assigned to this role.

When I was asking colleagues about why they were leaving the ICU, one nurse shared an experience that she had while shopping at Kmart. A store associate got on the overhead system to announce a "blue light special." For those of you who have never shopped at Kmart, a "blue light special" is typically an announcement made for a discounted price on an item for a limited amount of time and to in-store guests. The nurse was shopping when she heard the overhead announcement for a "blue light special," and she immediately panicked. She described that her heart was racing, and she couldn't catch her breath; for a moment, she thought she was in the ICU. Ultimately, she left the ICU and attributes it to this experience and others that caused similar reactions.

Another colleague that I talked with described increased anxiety when working in the ICU. What finally led to her leaving the ICU was a response she experienced whenever she drove to work. On her way to work, she would drive around a bend that would connect one highway to another. That connection meant that she was only about a mile from the hospital. Every time she approached that bend, without fail, she would have symptoms of a panic attack. She was trembling, having heart palpitations, and sweating, and felt sick to her stomach.

I could write an entire book with the countless stories I have heard from nurses. The point I'm trying to get across is that these nurses were my colleagues, and they were intelligent, skillful, and compassionate caregivers. They thrived in the ICU for many years, but eventually the emotional stress was too much for them to handle. It was these powerful and similar stories along with the PTSS-10 survey questions that led to my first research project in the area of provider wellness.

Our team initially looked at the prevalence of symptoms of PTSD, anxiety, depression, and burnout syndrome in critical care nurses compared to general medical-surgical nurses in a local university system. This was accomplished through a self-report questionnaire that included reliable and validated instruments. Interestingly, the prevalence of PTSD symptoms was high in both groups. In fact, the prevalence was similar to that of combat veterans returning from the war in Iraq and Afghanistan. To better address whether this high prevalence of distress was an institutional issue or a generalizable nursing issue, we administered the same questionnaire to nurses within a one-hundred-mile radius of our institution with similar results.

Next, we looked at the prevalence of PTSD, anxiety, depression, and burnout syndrome in nurses on a national level to better address generalizability. We hypothesized that we would continue to see high levels of distress. If this was true, we also wanted to know what to do about it. Organizational change takes time and would not eliminate all of the stresses inherent to taking care of acute or critically ill patients; therefore, we focused on the individual nurse and the ability of the individual nurse to adapt and thrive through personal practices. We introduced a measure of psychological resilience to this national sample of nurses to understand whether resilience impacted symptoms of psychological distress and healthy daily functioning for nurses at work and in their home environments (discussed in Chapter 3).

Finally, based on the results of our national study, we began developing and piloting promising behavioral resilience interventions to assess feasibility and acceptability in nurses. Do they like the interventions? Will they sustain a resilience practice after participation in a study? With busy schedules, are the nurses able to engage and complete the interventions? The pilot studies were also a way of generating preliminary data on whether resilience interventions were effective in improving resilience scores and mitigating symptoms of distress.

Within the last 5 years, professional organizations have started to take notice and assign priority to clinician wellbeing. If you pick up a peer-reviewed healthcare journal, there is almost always one article related to clinician distress and what to do about it. Nurses are not alone. Physicians, physical therapists, pharmacists, respiratory therapists, social works, and other acute care professionals are exposed to patient-related stressors and/or organization-related stressors that may cause distress. However, I would argue that cumulative and repeated exposure to distressing situations is unique to nursing, particularly in specialty areas such as the ICU where there is increased mortality and witnessing of unnatural and disturbing suffering that is often the consequence of caregiving. As nurses, we are trusted to care for others.

In fact, nurses continue to receive high marks for honesty and ethical standards, outscoring doctors, dentists, pharmacists, clergy, and police officers. Eighty-five percent of Americans give nursing "high" or "very high" scores, making it the most trusted profession in the United States for the 17th consecutive year (Gallup, 2018).

Why are nurses the most trusted profession...because we *care* about people and there is often a genuine connection because of that therapeutic relationship. Most people that you talk to will have a personal story about an experience they had with a nurse. That personal story may be an individual experience or an experience that a family member or loved one had with a nurse. In fact, a lot of times, that's what draws a person to the profession of nursing. In a survey of over 700 nurses in the United States, 67% reported entering the profession because they wanted to help and care for people (Mealer, 2012). As a caring profession, are nurses primed for the psychological consequences of the stressful work environment? There are tens of thousands of nurses in the United States alone that suffer both personally and professional from work-related stress. It is caring that draws individuals to the profession of nursing, but it is also what is driving nurses away from the profession. In this book, my goal is to provide education, awareness, and individual self-care practices that may be helpful to the individual nurse. Obviously, there are situations in the acute care environment that cannot be changed. Nurses are inherently exposed to patient suffering, death, and morally challenging decisions, but developing personal practices and skills better equips us for *coping with caring*.

References

Brenan, M. (2018). Nurses again outpace other professions for honesty, ethics. *Gallup*. Retrieved from: https://news.gallup.com/poll/245597/nurses-again-outpace-professions-honesty-ethics.aspx.

Mealer, M., Jones, J., Newman, J., McFann, K., Rothbaum, B. & Moss, M. (2012). The presence of resilience is associated with a healthier psychological profile in intensive care unit (ICU) nurses: Results of a national survey. *International Journal of Nursing Studies*, 49, 292–299.

Author

Meredith Mealer is an Associate Professor of Medicine in the Department of Physical Medicine and Rehabilitation at the University of Colorado Anschutz Medical Campus. She holds a PhD in nursing and has completed post-graduate work as a psychiatric mental health nurse practitioner. Prior to being at the University of Colorado, she worked in critical care for 12 years at Emory University Healthcare. She is a national and international expert on clinician distress as a result of the stressful work environment, and her primary area of research is resilience training and the various behavioral research interventions that can mitigate psychological distress in the workplace. Dr. Mealer is also the Director of Research for the Wellbeing Collaborative within the American Thoracic Society (ATS), which is a leadership team that is addressing burnout syndrome for pulmonary, sleep, and critical care healthcare providers. Additionally, she co-chaired the professional issues panel for the American Nurses Association (ANA) to develop policy and identify strategies to strengthen moral resilience within practicing nurses. This resulted in the call-to-action *Exploring Moral Resilience Toward a Culture of Ethical Practice.*

Chapter 1

Psychological
Distress in Nursing

Working as an acute care nurse is stressful. Let me say that again, working as an acute care nurse is *stressful*. The reason for the stress is multifactorial, but potential triggers or stressors include, but are not limited to, long 12-h shifts, high patient acuity, high patient mortality, interacting with verbally abusive family members or coworkers, ethical or moral dilemmas,

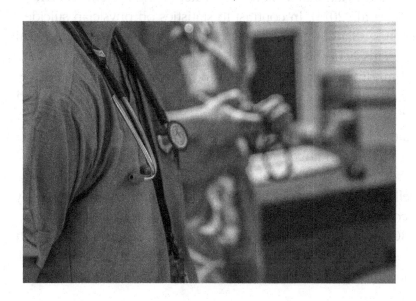

organizational policies, and staffing issues. Oftentimes, it is the combination and cumulative effect of these stressors that causes distress in nurses. There are nurses who are able to cope with the stress of working in the acute care environment, and this will be discussed in greater detail in Chapter 3. However, the prevalence of psychological distress is quite common in acute care nurses, which may lead to maladaptive responses such as sleeping difficulties, relationship issues, substance abuse, and suicide.

The incidence of suicide in physicians is well known because there are mechanisms in place to document death in this manner. It was recently reported that suicide was the leading cause of death in male residents and the second most prevalent cause of death in female residents (Yaghmour et al., 2017). This data is available on residents because the Accreditation Council for Graduate Medical Education (ACGME) maintains information on all U.S. accredited graduate medical education programs and specifically records deaths and cause of deaths in their Accreditation Data System (ADS) records. Approximately 300 U.S. physicians will die by suicide each year, which is available in the Centers for Disease Control and Prevention National Violent Death Reporting System (NVDRS) (Gold et al., 2013). In contrast to statistics on physician suicide, statistics related to nurse suicide in the United States are unavailable. This is unfortunate, as there would likely be resources and funding dedicated to instituting support systems geared toward suicide prevention in nursing. Data in England revealed that between the years 2011 and 2015, the risk of suicide among health professionals was 24% higher than the national average, and this was in large part because of the suicide rate among nurses, which was 23% above the national average (Windsor-Shellard, 2017). Additionally, nurses were four times more likely to commit suicide than people outside of the healthcare field (BBC News, 2000). The most common reason for the increased rate of suicide in both physicians and nurses is depression and other undiagnosed/untreated mental health conditions.

Psychological distress in nurses has also been associated with decreased quality of patient care, increased nosocomial infections, increased medication errors, increase in 30-day mortality rates, and decreased patient satisfaction (Cimiotti et al., 2012; Poghosyan, 2010).

What is meant by psychological distress? There are several concepts in the literature related to the distress experienced by nurses. Compassion fatigue, moral distress, secondary traumatic stress, and vicarious traumatization will be discussed below as symptoms or syndromes and if left untreated can lead to the development of psychological disorders such as anxiety, depression, burnout syndrome, and/or posttraumatic stress disorder (PTSD).

Compassion Fatigue/Secondary Traumatic Stress and Vicarious Traumatization

Compassion fatigue, secondary traumatic stress, and vicarious traumatization will be discussed together as they are often used interchangeably in the literature although each is from different theoretical underpinnings.

Compassion fatigue in nursing was first described over three decades ago and is a phenomenon specific to caregivers who help patients that have been traumatized. Joinson describes compassion fatigue as either a trigger or a consequence of burnout syndrome (1992) with the patient being exposed to the trauma and the nurse or caregiver experiencing the secondary effects of that trauma. Compassion fatigue in other caregiver groups has been described as a concept with a more positive connotation than secondary traumatic stress and vicarious traumatization (Adams, 2006). There is an increased prevalence of compassion fatigue in emergency room nurses, critical care nurses, hospice settings, oncology, mental health, nephrology, medical and surgical units, and pediatrics (Abendroth & Flannery, 2006;

Meadors & Lamson, 2008; Robins et al., 2009, Hooper et al., 2010; Potter et al., 2010, Yoder, 2010). Some nurses may decide to leave the profession or change the type of unit they are working in because of compassion fatigue, but many are able to maintain a healthy balance between the positive and negative attributes of caring. On the opposite end of the compassion fatigue spectrum is compassion satisfaction, which is the cumulative effects of the positive feelings a caregiver experiences as a result of helping others (Sacco et al., 2015).

Secondary traumatic stress is a phenomenon similar to compassion fatigue as described above and is caused by a nurse's interaction with trauma victims, which is also classified as being indirectly traumatized due to witnessing trauma to another individual. It has been described as the development of PTSD in healthcare providers. Interestingly, measures of secondary traumatic stress include the three symptom clusters of PTSD: re-experiencing the event, hyperarousal symptoms, and symptoms of avoidance. The only areas missing for a diagnosis of PTSD are the endorsement of a specific traumatic event, how the event and symptoms affect daily functioning and the length of time the individual has been experiencing the event.

The prevalence of secondary traumatic stress in nurses ranges from 25% to 78% and has been reported in trauma, critical care, oncology, forensic, and hospice nurses.

Vicarious Traumatization was introduced as a concept in 1990 by McCann & Pearlman to describe altered cognitions and memory imagery systems experienced by mental health therapists who experience prolonged exposure to the traumatic experiences of their patients. The underlying mechanism of vicarious traumatization is thought to be countertransference or the therapist's unresolved conflicts outside of the therapeutic relationship, which interferes with their ability to distinguish their patient's trauma from their own personal traumas (McCann & Pearlman, 1990). As with secondary traumatic stress, the symptoms of vicarious traumatization include the

PTSD symptoms clusters of re-experiencing the event, hyper-arousal, and avoidance. Trauma counselors and counselors in sexual abuse and assault experienced changes in their belief system and sense of identity as a result of working with this population of traumatized individuals (Collins & Long, 2003).

Moral Distress

Moral distress is a complex concept, and definitions vary considerably. Jameton's definition states that moral distress occurs "when the nurse makes a moral judgment about a case in which or he is involved and the institution or coworkers make it difficult or impossible for the nurse to act on that judgment" (Jameton, 1993). Moral distress occurs when there is a need for a morally responsible action, a strategy is determined by the nurse based on individual moral beliefs and the nurse is unable to institute their strategy or action plan due to internal or external constraints. Repeated exposure to ethical dilemmas may illicit more intense symptoms due to recalling earlier stressful situations. The consequences of moral distress include burnout syndrome, depression, anxiety, and ultimately turnover of experienced bedside nurses. Nurses are most at risk for moral distress compared with physicians due to perceptions that they are unable to make decisions during morally complex conversations (Rushton, 2016; Moss et al., 2016; Mealer & Moss, 2016). Up to 80% of nurses experience symptoms of moral distress with the highest prevalence among critical care nurses. Clinical situations that may cause symptoms of moral distress include futile treatments, inappropriate care, inadequate pain relief, incompetent coworkers, hastening the dying process, and providing false hope (Moss et al., 2016).

The next sections will discuss the consequences of moral distress, vicarious traumatization, secondary traumatic stress, and compassion fatigue, which includes burnout syndrome and PTSD.

Burnout Syndrome

Burnout syndrome isn't new. In fact, the concept has been around for several decades. First described in the late 1970s and early 1980s, burnout syndrome has universally involved a state of fatigue or emotional exhaustion that is caused by prolonged job stress. Depending on the philosophical or existential perspective, burnout syndrome may also include characteristics such as the failure to produce an expected goal, a syndrome that develops from long-term involvement in emotionally demanding situations or a concept that is a direct result of "people work" and, together with emotional exhaustion, results in depersonalization and/or a reduced sense of personal accomplishment (Freudenberg & Richelson, 1980; Pines & Aronson, 1988; Maslach, 1982).

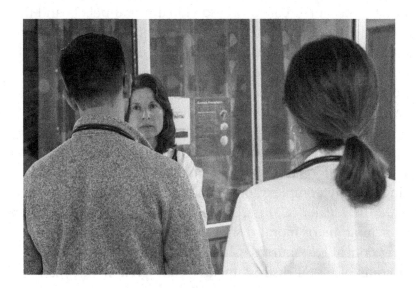

The definition of burnout syndrome was born out of pragmatic concerns instead of theoretical and academic inquiry; the concept was stretched to involve almost all personal problems; and burnout syndrome was largely non-empirical during its early stages of development. These issues have caused confusion and debate in the academic world as the concept of burnout syndrome in healthcare professionals has taken center stage. Professional societies and organizations over the past few years have started to appreciate the pervasive nature of burnout syndrome in the nursing workforce and are trying to understand the impact of burnout syndrome on the individual provider's mental health, turnover of experienced staff, and patient outcome consequences. The issues being debated include the definition or conceptualization of burnout syndrome, and how burnout syndrome is measured and/or diagnosed in the nursing population, and more broadly the healthcare provider population.

Defining Burnout Syndrome in Nursing

Again, as described above, the concept of burnout syndrome did not arise from a theoretical perspective. Originally, burnout syndrome was defined through a social psychology and psychiatry lens to describe a depletion of emotion and lost motivation and commitment observed in the workplace. The most commonly adopted definition of burnout syndrome in healthcare and nursing is Maslach's (1982) definition that states "burnout is a syndrome of emotional exhaustion, depersonalization, and a reduced personal accomplishment that can occur among individuals who do 'people work' of some kind" (Maslach). In nursing, burnout syndrome has been described as involving common organizational workplace triggers but also trauma and stress triggers, which may overlap with anxiety, depression, and PTSD.

Triggers of Burnout Syndrome in Nursing

In a recent qualitative study that was conducted to design a resilience intervention for critical care nurses to reduce burnout syndrome, nurses from around the United States were asked to provide examples of specific triggers that caused burnout syndrome. The triggers would be used to design didactic content and begin to train nurses to address these triggers with resilience mechanisms instead of maladaptive coping skills. The triggers were categorized as environmental, administrative, and psychological. The environmental triggers identified included working with inexperienced nurses, coworker apathy, family needs, fast turnover of patients, staffing issues, and mandatory overtime. Administrative triggers involved inadequate training, environments not conducive to learning, interdepartmental/intradepartmental arguments among coworkers, no regard to staff cohesiveness when trying to fill a full-time nursing position, and administrations apparent disconnect with the issues of bedside nurses. Finally, the psychological triggers involved anxiety from being the most experienced nurse on the unit, guilt associated with "bad care," emotional injury, startle reactions to monitor alarms, and not having time to debrief or grieve after a patient death (Mealer, 2017). Identifying these triggers is also important to better understand whether burnout syndrome in nursing is a distinct and unique concept as compared to burnout

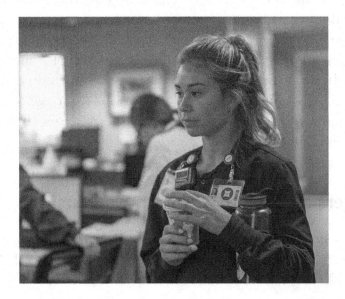

syndrome in other healthcare personnel. In contrast, should burnout syndrome be differentiated from the concurrent development of psychological disorders such as anxiety, depression, and PTSD?

Measuring and Diagnosing Burnout Syndrome in Nursing

There are several measures of burnout syndrome that have limited application to the nursing population. The two most common and applicable measures in nursing include the Burnout Measure (BM) (Pines & Aronson, 1988) and the Maslach Burnout Inventory Health Services Survey (MBI-HSS) (Maslach & Jackson, 1981). Additionally, these measures have the most robust psychometric analyses.

The Burnout Measure

The BM is based on the definition of burnout syndrome as "a state of physical, emotional and mental exhaustion caused by long-term involvement in situations that are emotionally demanding" (Pines & Aronson, 1988). There are 21 items scored on a 7-point rating scale from "never" to always," and the psychometric testing has been conducted in 30 different samples and 3,900 subjects with a coefficient alpha of 0.91–0.93.

The Maslach Burnout Inventory

The MBI is the most commonly used measure of burnout syndrome in all disciplines. The MBI was developed and based on Maslach's definition as written above. The MBI is a 22-item survey with three independently scored dimensions (emotional exhaustion, depersonalization, and a reduced sense of personal accomplishment), on a 7-point Likert scale. Psychometric analyses have been completed on over 11,000 subjects from many different populations with a coefficient alpha of 0.71–0.90.

There is question concerning whether the MBI is a valid instrument to use in the nursing population. Adequate coefficient alpha scores represent the reliability of an instrument or consistent results over time. Validity refers to the ability of an instrument to measure what is intended to be measured and is based on the definition and theoretical underpinning of the concept. An exploratory and confirmatory factor analysis of the MBI-HSS in nurses indicated a two-factor model had the best fit indices and fifteen of the original questions were removed based on factor loadings (Schneider et al., 2018). Therefore, since the MBI-HSS is the most commonly used burnout inventory in nursing and the validity of the instrument is questionable in its current form, it is most likely not measuring what it claims to measure.

Self-report instruments are used as quick screening procedures to determine whether symptoms associated with a condition are present and whether a more in-depth interview is needed to diagnose a condition. Aside from the questions of how to conceptualize and identify burnout syndrome in nursing is whether there are specific diagnostic criteria for burnout.

Diagnosing Burnout Syndrome

There is paucity of information related to the diagnosis of burnout syndrome. Bibeau et al. (1989), based on an analysis of the various definitions proposed both subjective and objective diagnostic criteria. The subjective factors included self-determination of severe fatigue that is accompanied by problems concentrating, irritability, and negativism; physical symptoms of distress without a medical cause; and a loss of self-esteem. The objective factors include assessments by the healthcare provider's patients, supervisors, and colleagues that imply a significant decrease in work performance over a period of several months. The most interesting caveat to these criteria states that the subjective and objective factors should not result from the healthcare provider not being competent (or a novice provider), the absence of major psychopathology (such as depression, anxiety, and PTSD), and should not be related to outside influences such as family-related problems. In addition, despite these specific diagnostic criteria, a separate Diagnostic and Statistical Manual of Mental Disorders, Version 5 (DSM-V) diagnostic category would be unnecessary because it could be included as a subcategory of an adjustment disorder with work inhibition (Bibeau et al., 1989; Schaufeli et al., 2008).

Regardless of the concerns about definition, conceptualization, measurement, and diagnosis, burnout syndrome remains a significant concern in nursing.

Prevalence of Burnout Syndrome in Nursing

There have been multiple studies to report the prevalence of burnout syndrome in nurses, and the results suggest that approximately 30% manifest symptoms of severe burnout syndrome and up to 86% are positive for at least one of the subscales of burnout as defined by Maslach (emotional exhaustion, depersonalization, and a reduced sense of personal accomplishment) (Embriaco et al., 2007; Poncet et al., 2007; Mealer et al., 2009, 2012; Patrick & Lavery, 2007; Epp, 2012). The prevalence of burnout is not significantly higher based on the nurses work environment; however, there is a higher prevalence of burnout syndrome and concurrent PTSD diagnoses/symptoms in nurses that work in high-stress environments including critical care, bone marrow transplant unit, high-risk obstetrics unit, post-operative anesthesia unit (PACU), operating room, and emergency department (Mealer et al., 2009).

Posttraumatic Stress Disorder

PTSD is classified as a trauma-and-stressor-related disorder, which explicitly includes exposure to a traumatic or stressful event. The criteria needed for a diagnosis of PTSD include (a) exposure to a traumatic event (i.e., direct exposure, witnessing the event, learning of an event that happened to a close friend or family member, and repeated exposure to aversive details of a traumatic event), (b) presence of one or more intrusion symptoms (i.e., recurrent, non-volitional memories of the event, nightmares, dissociation), (c) avoidance of reminders of the traumatic event (i.e., places, people, thoughts), (d) negative cognitions and mood associated with event, (e) hypervigilance or sleep disturbances, (f) a duration of symptoms for at least 1 month, (g) clinically significant disturbances in important areas of functioning, and (h) the symptoms and functional impairments are not the result of substance abuse or another medical condition (DSM-V, 2013).

PTSD in Nursing

Nurses are exposed to traumatic events in the work environment. This may be through direct exposure, witnessing a traumatic event happening to a patient, or repeated exposure to aversive details of a traumatic event (see Table 1.1 for potential examples of each).

Theoretical Perspective of PTSD in Nursing

The development of PTSD is dose dependent. This means that individuals who have been exposed to one traumatic event are at an increased risk for developing PTSD after a subsequent exposure. It is hypothesized that prior exposure to a traumatic event sensitizes individuals to respond with

Table 1.1   Traumatic Exposures

Trauma Exposure/ Direct Exposure	Trauma Exposure/ Witnessing Trauma	Trauma Exposure/ Repeated Exposure
Physical or verbal abuse by patients	Seeing patients die	Postmortem care and handling of dead bodies
Physical or verbal abuse by family members	Performing "futile" and oftentimes painful care	Stress related to not being able to save a specific patient
Physical or verbal abuse by coworkers/ ancillary staff	Caring for patients with traumatic injuries	Repeated involvement with end-of-life care
Infectious body fluid splash to the eyes or mouth	Performing cardiopulmonary resuscitation	Emotional injury related to death and dying
Infectious needle stick	Massive hemorrhaging	Guilt associated with "bad care"

more intensity to subsequent events (Cougle et al., 2009; Yehuda et al., 1995). The Nurse as Wounded Healer theory recognizes that *all* nurses experience both personal and professional trauma and suggests coping skills to ameliorate symptoms of trauma in order to prevent subsequent development of PTSD (Conti-O'Hare, 2002). We understand that there are organizational/institutional factors that contribute to burnout syndrome, psychological distress, and PTSD, but this theoretical perspective explores individual factors and coping skills that promote self-healing, allows transformation and transcendence of traumatic experiences, and ultimately prepares the nurse to use his/her experiences to therapeutically care for patients. The inability to self-heal through individual coping skills stymies these efforts, which can lead to the development of PTSD as well as changes in worldview, guilt and regret associated with nursing care, difficulty sleeping, and other functional outcomes (Mealer & Jones,

2013). Nurses are at an increased risk and vulnerable to PTSD considering the cumulative and dose-dependent attributes of trauma. This model of PTSD in nursing is shown in Figure 1.1.

Prevalence of PTSD Symptoms and Diagnosis in Nursing

In the United States, there is an 8%–10% lifetime prevalence of PTSD in the general population, and it is the fourth most common psychiatric disorder (Mealer et al., 2009; Yehuda, 2002). Unlike burnout syndrome, the prevalence of PTSD varies depending on the work environment of the nurse.

Fourteen percent of general medical-surgical nurses were positive for symptoms of PTSD compared to 24%–30% of

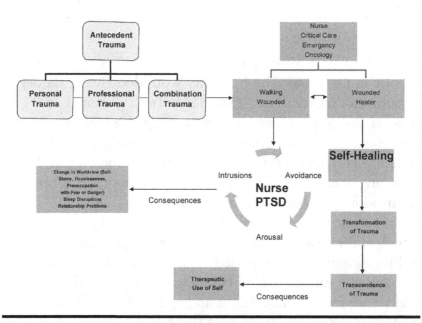

Figure 1.1 Model of nurse posttraumatic stress disorder. (Copyright © 2013. Used by permission of Wiley Periodicals, Inc. Nursing Forum, Volume 48, All rights reserved.)

intensive care unit (ICU) nurses ($p = 0.03$). ICU nurses also endorsed nightmares and anxiety or panic related to their experience working as a nurse (Mealer et al., 2007). It is difficult to determine the incidence of PTSD in nursing because the gold-standard diagnostic criteria include a clinically administered interview. However, the posttraumatic diagnostic scale (PDS) has an advantage of other self-report measures. The PDS is considered a diagnostic tool and meets all the DSM-V criteria for a diagnosis of PTSD. This tool has correlated well with the Clinically Administered PTSD Scale for DSM-5 (CAPS-5), and is well validated and reliable (Foa et al., 1997; Mealer et al., 2009). Based on the PDS, 5% of outpatient nurses, 18% of inpatient nurses outside of high-stress units, 22% of nurses in non-ICU high-stress units, and 23% of nurses in the ICU meet the diagnostic criteria for PTSD (Mealer et al., 2009). Of those nurses who met criteria for a PTSD diagnosis, there was significant impairment in functioning outside of work. Seventy-six percent endorsed problems with general satisfaction in life and 64% stated that it affected their overall level of functioning in all areas of their life (Mealer et al., 2009).

Overlap in Psychological Distress and/or Disorders in Nursing

As presented above, there is significant overlap between moral distress, compassion fatigue, secondary traumatic stress, vicarious traumatization, and PTSD. Moral distress, compassion fatigue, secondary traumatic stress, and vicarious traumatization address some of the criteria for a diagnosis of PTSD, which includes measuring symptoms of intrusion, avoidance, and hyperarousal (Mealer & Jones, 2013). What's missing is labeling a specific event as causing the trauma, the length of time that symptoms have been present, and how daily functioning has been affected by the trauma.

There is also overlap between burnout syndrome and PTSD with PTSD being a more severe subset of those with burnout syndrome. When comparing nurses with both burnout syndrome and a diagnosis of PTSD with nurses only exhibiting burnout syndrome, nurses with both burnout and PTSD were significantly more likely to have impairment in functioning (see Table 1.2).

Table 1.2   Effects on Life Outside of the Hospital in Nurses with Both PTSD and Burnout Syndrome Alone Compared with Nurses with Burnout Syndrome Alone (Percentage with Positive Response)

	Nurses with Both BOS and Diagnosis of PTSD	Nurses with BOS But No Diagnosis of PTSD	
	(n = 59)	*(n = 217)*	**P** *Value*
Household chores and duties	51%	22%	<0.0001
Relationships with friends	58%	16%	<0.0001
Fun and leisure activities	54%	20%	<0.0001
Schoolwork	15%	3%	0.001
Relationships with their family	49%	17%	<0.0001
Sex life	53%	16%	<0.0001
General satisfaction in life	76%	25%	<0.0001
Overall level of functioning in all areas of their life	64%	16%	<0.0001

Source: Copyright © 2009. Used by permission of Wiley Periodicals, Inc. Depression and Anxiety, Volume 26. All rights reserved.

BOS, burnout syndrome.

References

Adams, R., Boscarino, J. & Figley, C. (2006). Compassion fatigue and psychological distress among social workers: A validation study. *American Journal of Orthopsychiatry*, 76, 103–108.

Abendroth, M. & Flannery, J. (2006). Predicting the risk of compassion fatigue: A study of hospice nurses. *Journal of Hospice and Palliative Nursing*, 8, 346–356.

American Psychological Association (2013). *Diagnostic and Statistical Manual of Mental Disorders*, 5th edition. Washington, DC: American Psychiatric Publishing.

BBC News (2000). 'Suicide Risk' for doctors and nurses. Retrieved from: www.news.bbc.co,uk/2/hi/health/944503.stm

Bibeau, G., Dussault, G., Larouche, L.M., Lippel, K.I., Saucier, J.F., Vezina, M. & Vidal, J.M. (1989). *Some Cultural Diagnostic and Juridical Aspects of Burnout*. Monreal: Confedration des Syndicats Nationaux.

Cimiotti, J.P., Aiken, L.H., Sloane, D.M. & Wu, E.S. (2012). Nurse staffing, burnout, and health care-associated infection. *American Journal of Infection Control*, 40, 486–490.

Collins, S. & Long, A. (2003). Working with the psychological effects of trauma: Consequences for mental health-care workers-a literature review. *Journal of Psychiatric Mental Health Nursing*, 10, 417–424.

Conti-O'Hare, M. (2002). *The Nurse as Wounded Healer: From Trauma to Transcendence*. Sudbury, MA: Jones and Bartlett.

Cougle, J., Resnick, H. & Kilpatrick, D. (2009). Does prior exposure to interpersonal violence increase risk of PTSD following subsequent exposure? *Behaviour Research and Therapy*, 47, 1012–1017.

Embriaco, N., Papazian, L., Kentish-Barnes, N., Pochard, F. & Azoulay, E. (2007). Burnout syndrome among critical care healthcare workers. *Current Opinion in Critical Care*, 13, 482–488.

Epp, K. (2012). Burnout in critical care nurses: A literature review. *Dynamics*, 23, 25–31.

Foa, E., Cashman, L., Jaycox, L & Perry, K. (1997). The validation of a self-report measure of posttraumatic stress disorder. The posttraumatic diagnostic scale. *Psychological Assessment*, 9(4), 445–451.

Freudenberger, H. & Richelson, G. (1980). Burn-out: Occupational hazard of the child care worker. *Child Care Quarterly*, 6, 90–99.

Gold, K.J., Sen, A. & Schwenk, T.L. (2013). Detail on suicide among US physicians: Data from the National Violent Death Reporting System. *General Hospital Psychiatry*, 35, 45–49.

Hooper, C., Craig, J., Janvrin, D.R., Wetsel, M.A. & Reimels, E. (2010). Compassion satisfaction, burnout, and compassion fatigue among emergency nurses compared with nurses in other selected inpatient specialties. *Journal of Emergency Nursing*, 36, 420–427.

Jameton, A. (1993). Dilemmas of moral distress: Moral responsibility and nursing practice. *Clinical Issues in Perinatal Women's Health Nursing*, 4, 542–551.

Joinson, C. (1992). Coping with compassion fatigue. *Nursing*, 116, 118–119.

Maslach, C. & Jackson, S. (1981). The measurement of experienced burnout. *Journal of Organizational Behavior*, 2, 99–113.

Maslach, C. (1982). Understanding burnout: Definitional issues in analyzing a complex phenomenon. In W.S. Paine (Ed.), *Job Stress and Burnout* (pp. 29–40). Beverly Hills, CA: Sage.

McCann, L. & Pearlman, L. (1990). Vicarious traumatization: A framework for understanding the psychological effects of working with victims. *Journal of Traumatic Stress*, 3(1), 131–149.

Meadors, P. & Lamson, A. (2008). Compassion fatigue and secondary traumatization: Provider self care on intensive care units for children. *Journal of Pediatric Health Care*, 22(1), 24–34.

Mealer, M., Shelton, A., Berg, B., Rothbaum, B. & Moss, M. (2007). Increased prevalence of post-traumatic stress disorder symptoms in critical care nurses. *American Journal of Respiratory & Critical Care Medicine*, 175, 693–697.

Mealer, M., Burnham, E., Goode, C.J., Rothbaum, B. & Moss, M. (2009). The prevalence and Impact of post traumatic stress disorder and burnout syndrome in nurses. *Depression and Anxiety*, 26, 1118–1126.

Mealer, M., Jones, J., Newman, J., McFann, K.K., Rothbaum, B. & Moss, M. (2012). The presence of resilience is associated with a healthier psychological profile in intensive care unit (ICU) nurses: Results of a national survey. *International Journal of Nursing Studies*, 49, 292–299.

Mealer, M. & Jones, J. (2013). Posttraumatic stress disorder in the nursing population: A concept Analysis. *Nursing Forum*, 48, 279–288.

Mealer, M. & Moss, M. (2016). Moral distress in ICU nurses. *Intensive Care Medicine*, 42(10), 1615–1617.

Mealer, M., Hodapp, R., Conrad, D., Dimidjian, S., Rothbaum, B. & Moss, M. (2017). Designing a resilience program for critical care nurses. *AACN Advanced Critical Care*, 28, 359-365.

Moss, M., Good, V., Gozal, D., Kleinpell, R. & Sessler, C. (2016). A critical care collaborative statement: Burnout syndrome in critical care health-care professionals. A call for action. *American Journal of Respiratory & Critical Care Medicine*, 194(1), 106–113.

Patrick, K. & Lavery, J.F. (2007). Burnout in nursing. *Australian Journal of Advanced Nursing*, 24, 43–48.

Pines, A. & Aronson, E. (1988). *Career Burnout: Causes and Cures*. New York: Free Press.

Poghosyan, L., Clarke, S.P., Finlayson, M. & Aiken, L.H. (2010). Nurse burnout and quality of care: cross-national investigation in six countries. *Research in Nursing & Health*, 33, 288–298.

Poncet, M.C., Toullic, P., Papazian, L., Kentish-Barnes, N., Timsit, J.F., Pochard, F., Chevret, S., Schlemmer, B. & Azoulay, E. (2007). Burnout syndrome in critical care nursing staff. *American Journal of Respiratory & Critical Care Medicine*, 175, 698–704.

Potter, P., Deshields, T., Divanbeigi, J., Berger, J., Cipriano, D., Norris, L., Olsen, S. (2010). Compassion fatigue and burnout: Prevalence among oncology nurses. *Clinical Journal of Oncology Nursing*, 14, 56–62.

Robins, P.M., Meltzer, L. & Zelikovsky, N. (2009). The experience of secondary traumatic stress upon care providers working within a children's hospital. *Journal of Pediatric Nursing*, 24, 270–279.

Rushton, C.H. (2016). Moral resilience: A capacity for navigating moral distress in critical care. *AACN Advanced Critical Care*, 27, 111–119.

Sacco, T., Ciurzynski, S., Harvey, M. & Ingersoll, G. (2015). Compassion satisfaction and compassion fatigue among critical care nurses. *Critical Care Nurse*, 35, 32–43.

Schaufeli, W., Leiter, M. & Maslach, C. (2008). Burnout: 35 years of research and practice. *Career Development International*, 14, 204–220.

Schneider, A., Forster, J. & Mealer, M. (in press). Exploratory and confirmatory factor analysis of the Maslach Burnout Inventory to Measure Burnout Syndrome in Critical Care Nurses, *Journal of Nursing Measurement*. Accepted on November 10, 2018.

Windsor-Shellard, B. (2017). Suicide by occupation, England: 2011 to 2015. Office for National Statistics.

Yaghmour, N., Brigham, T., Richter, T., Miller, R., Philiber, I., Baldwin, D. & Nasca, T. (2017). Causes of death of residents in ACGME accredited programs 2000–2014: Implications for the learning environment, Academic Medicine, 92, 976–983. www.ons.gov.uk/peoplepopulationandcommunity/birthsdeathsandmarriages/deaths/articles/suicidebyoccupation/england2011to2015.

Yehuda, R., Kaahana, B., Schmeidler, J., Southwick, S., Wilson, S. & Giller, E. (1995). Impact Of cumulative lifetime trauma and recent stress on current posttraumatic stress disorder symptoms in holocaust survivors. *American Journal of Psychiatry*, 152, 1815–1818.

Yehuda, R. (2002). Posttraumatic stress disorder. *The New England Journal of Medicine*, 346, 108–114.

Yoder, E.A. (2010). Compassion fatigue in nurses. *Applied Nursing Research*, 23, 191–197.

Chapter 2

Triggers and Narratives

Psychological stress and the ability to cope with that stress can be quite challenging for nurses. Unlike other professions outside of healthcare, nurses' face a variety of environmental and patient-related experiences that, through cumulative exposure, serve as triggers and/or catalysts to the development of symptoms related to common psychological disorders, as discussed in Chapter 1.

Environmental triggers that have been identified as contributors to stress include mandatory overtime, long work hours, fast turnover of patients, coworker arguments/pettiness, inadequate training for advanced technical procedures, staffing issues, and navigating high acuity patient loads in a unit with new, inexperienced nurses. It is difficult to understand the impact of these triggers and convey the emotion that nurses experience because of these triggers, through text alone. So, instead of providing a description of these triggers within the lens of nursing, I will share powerful personal narratives that nurse participants shared during a pilot research study on the use of written exposure therapy (WET) to build resilience and reduce symptoms associated with burnout syndrome, posttraumatic stress disorder (PTSD), anxiety, and depression. The use of writing therapy as a resilience intervention and coping mechanism will be discussed in Chapter 5.

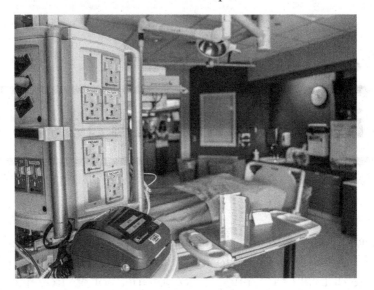

Junior Nurses

Narrative #1

I had just recently gotten off orientation as a new graduate RN. I had only had 6 weeks to work with another RN before I was on my own and expected to know what to do. A patient came up and he sounded fairly sick, but I really didn't worry too much about it. The emergency department came up and put him in our bed and then left pretty quickly. They were probably busy that night, but it was really annoying to me that they had dumped and run.

The certified nursing assistant (CNA) and I were getting the patient settled and talking to him and his wife. He WAS talking, I'm almost positive, but now, I have started to doubt myself and this detail. We couldn't get a blood pressure with the machine, and we couldn't get an O_2 saturation reading. I sent the CNA to get a manual cuff and an ear probe but didn't think too much about either of these things. I wasn't too worried and yet looking back these should have been my first clues that this patient wasn't doing well. I blame myself for missing this. I often wonder if it would have made a difference and if I could have saved him. This is why I doubt that I actually talked to him. Did I really talk to him? Did I really have cause not to be worried? If you can talk to a person, at least you know they are somewhat ok. But did I really hear his voice or was I just moving through trying to get him settled and not paying enough attention to him, to his condition, was I not vigilant enough?

This is why I doubt my capabilities as a nurse now...I miss things still. Four years later, shouldn't I be better than I was as a new graduate? Am I a detriment to patients? I remember that the CNA hadn't come back yet and I asked a question that he didn't answer...I looked back and his eyes were wide and unseeing, a bit glazed. He wasn't moving. I'm not sure how long it took me to figure out what was happening but looking back it feels like it was too long. Instead of jumping into action, I went out of the room to grab the charge nurse. Honestly, I didn't know what to do. I should have known what to do and I had no clue. I felt a bit frozen just staring at him knowing he was in trouble, but I was unable to help him. I come back to this moment a lot during cardiac arrests or patient resuscitations. Sometimes, I feel paralyzed...I know I should help but I just don't know how. If you asked me any other time, I could give you a detailed step-by-step guide, but in the moment, I'm too scared to move or act like I already know I can't help them and they are already lost. I want someone else to come in and help, to give me instructions, to be responsible. The charge nurse called a Medical Emergency Team (MET)—he was still gasping for breath and had a weak pulse, and his wife said he was a do not resuscitate (DNR), so I guess I didn't fail too badly because it isn't like there was much we could have done anyway. Telemetry called me to say he was tachycardic and then very bradycardic... and I just hung up on her. I couldn't deal with her and this dying man.

Respiratory Therapy (RT) got there and started bagging him because gasping isn't a helpful breathing pattern. We tried NARCAN and other meds to bring him back, but eventually, he just lost a pulse and we couldn't do CPR (cardiopulmonary resuscitation). I felt so helpless, I felt so guilty, I felt useless, I felt angry with the emergency department for abandoning us. He just looked into space with his eyes wide and it took me a while to close them because I just stared at him, not knowing what to do. I went out to where the doctor was talking to his wife and she broke down and fell to the floor crying. I comforted her as best I could. Mostly just said how sorry I was and put a hand on her shoulder. I couldn't fix it. I stayed for as long as I could before I felt the emotions hit me like a wave. I was losing it and I had to get out of there. I went to the lounge and sobbed. I cried for him and for me. I was heartbroken that I had lost my first patient and I was angry with myself for not at least being competent.

After the wife left I didn't even know how to clean up his body. I had to get help again…I couldn't even do that for him on my own. Recently, another one of my patients coded again, in front of me and I just hit the button. I didn't grab the Ambu bag to start ventilating him and I didn't check for a pulse. I just called for help and then froze. I stood there calling his name as if I could wake him with just my voice… exactly how I reacted that first time. It's like a sick pattern that my brain is in and can't get out of. Like a dream where I can't really control my actions. I'm just watching it all happen. I want to help, I know what to do, why can't I get my hands to just MOVE.

I guess I feel a bit like being a nurse is like trying to control an out-of-control car. As soon as a shift starts you hit the ground running and things pop out of nowhere and you just try to hold on and keep things together. You just grab the wheel and try to steer as best you can until it's over and you go home. You are just holding on and hoping that no one ends up dying on your shift unless they are comfort care and you don't have to resuscitate them. You do your best to keep from pummeling anyone who gets in your way.

Narrative #2

About a year ago, I was a brand-new employee on the step-down unit. While I had been nurse for 2 years at another hospital, I felt in over my head coming to the step-down unit. I quickly learned that step-down consisted of very sick patients. This patient population was all new to me. Coming to the step-down unit, I was introduced to advanced post-operative patients, drips I had never heard of, and many lines/tubes/drains I had never even heard of. One of my first shifts, I was precepting along with a nurse that had been on the step-down unit for 5 years. We had a patient a few hours post-operative from getting a new pacemaker. The patient had completed her time of post-procedural bedrest and asked to go to the bathroom. I had escorted the patient seamlessly as she was young and of good health aside from her reason for admission, which was symptomatic bradycardia. As the patient was using the restroom, she suddenly said "I don't feel well," slouched over, and was slow to respond. Luckily, the patient's daughter was a nurse and laying on the couch sleeping. I yelled for assistance, but her daughter was the only one in sight. Her daughter stood with her in the bathroom and held her up so she didn't collapse on the floor as I yelled for other staff members. As staff came in, we were able to carry her to the bed, give her fluids, and stabilize her. I remember being very nervous and out of my element in this situation. I was unfamiliar with post-operative pacemaker patients, I was unfamiliar with working night shift and not having as many staff members around within a yelling distance. I also thought about if this patient's daughter was not in the room, I didn't know how I would get in touch with any other help. I had a Sysco phone in my pocket but was not familiar with any numbers to call. I also remember feeling abandoned that many preceptors assumed I knew what I was doing with these patients as I was an experienced nurse, despite the multiple times I said I was uncomfortable with the patient population.

Coworker Arguments

I was in the Navy for 8 years prior to being a nurse, and I tend to have a very strong personality. I take my job as a nurse very seriously, and I like to joke around as well. The stressful situation I encountered was when my charge nurse/mentor told me I have had multiple complaints from coworkers saying that I'm too cocky and I don't take this job seriously. That was very hurtful to me because no one has ever said anything to my face about this. It also came to me as a surprise because I'm consistently getting positive feedback from my patients. This is stressful for me, because now when I come to work, I have a hard time trusting anyone. Are the people in my hall today the ones that are talking about me behind my back? Can I ask these people for help? I actually was coming around the corner when I heard one of my old preceptors saying to another coworker "he's been off lately" because I'm quieter and more reserved now.

In the military, I could count on anyone giving me feedback to my face so we can all grow together. In nursing, I feel like everyone is out for themselves at times. This hasn't always been the case on the unit. When I first was on my own from being a new graduate nurse on the unit, everyone was very helpful and friendly. They would invite me out to have a beer, and the camaraderie was evident. Now, it is just the girls on the unit always having girls' night out. It's hard because my wife and I don't have a lot of friends here because we moved here from out of State. Ever since my charge nurse brought this information to my knowledge, I have had a real tough time wanting to go to work. I'm actually applying for graduate school because I feel like maybe bedside nursing is just not for me. I'm passionate about what I do, and I enjoy having patients to take care of, but my coworkers can definitely make me feel very small. I've also been trying to take on more leadership roles, which I've been passed up on because of these complaints. I'm just not sure what I'm supposed to do at this point. I used to get bombs lobbed at our base in Afghanistan, and some days, I'd rather be back there than have coworkers that are supposed to have my back talk about me in secret. I try to drop everything at the door when I leave the hospital, but some days, it wears on me. One thing that I don't do is bring any negative emotions into my patient's room. I realize I have to be 100% strong and reliable for my patients because they are in their most vulnerable state. When I'm around my coworkers, even the ones that I've considered friends, I have my guard up. This has definitely been a learning experience for the last 6 months.

Patient Deaths

Narrative #1

I had a left ventricular assist device (LVAD) patient when I was a new graduate that I became very attached to. At first, I had trouble finding connection with this patient because I didn't know him very well and I was intimidated by the relationship the other nurses had with him. It was after many, many visits of taking care of him that I felt that there was a more comfortable sort of bond developing. The patient kept being admitted for bleeding problems and nonspecific abdominal pain and complaints that his pump "just didn't feel right." We kept admitting him, doing a workup, finding nothing wrong on his labs or tests, and then sending him home. He was probably admitted six to seven times over a 5–6-week period, and I took care of him each time and got to know he and his wife very well. His last admission was the same thing. He came in complaining that he just didn't feel right, we couldn't find any-thing wrong with him, and ended up discharging him, which he wanted because he was sick of being in the hospital.

Two days later, we heard that his wife was on her way to the hospital with him (LVAD patients are often driven by their families because EMS (Emergency Medical Service(s)) staff are too unfamiliar with their pumps). I began getting a room ready for him and stocking it with the equipment that would be needed. An hour later, we heard that the patient was in the emergency department, but was going to go to the intensive care unit (ICU). I asked our nurse practitioner (NP) if she knew why he was going to the ICU and she said that she didn't know specifically, but the emergency department had called and said the patient was unresponsive. She was sprint-ing toward the elevator to go see the patient when she told me this. My coworkers and I waited anxiously to hear any news, and after about an hour and a half, our cardiologist and NP came back to our unit and resumed rounding on patients. I asked our cardiologist if he had fixed the patient and he said "we're trying," which confused me since he was not down in the ICU with the patient. I asked permission from my charge nurse to go down and see the patient in the ICU. When I got down there, I decided just to go see the patient's wife in the waiting room so I wouldn't get in the way of the ICU nurses and their treatment. I saw one of our chaplains sitting with the patient's wife and realized that the situation must be much more serious than I thought. I gave his wife a big hug and asked if the ICU had told her anything. She said that all of his labs were out of whack and they had just started him on continuous renal replacement therapy (CRRT), which is a last resort for the kidneys. She was tearful, but seemed more shaken up than scared. I gave her another hug, told her I had to go back upstairs, but that we were all praying for them.

Two hours later, we got a call that the patient had died. This was a huge shock to me. Up to that point, I had viewed our ICU doctors and cardiologists as almost all powerful.

We had never lost an LVAD patient unexpectedly like this. I went down to the ICU after my shift to say goodbye to the patient. I went to his room and found the ICU nurses performing postmortem care. I began crying. Prior to this, I had never cried over a patient and prided myself on that. Seeing that patient exposed, looking like the same man I had just discharged 2 days ago was a shock. I then went to the waiting room and found his wife there. She saw me coming from across the room and immediately stood up to give me a hug as we wept together. I had never built such a close bond with a patient before or since. I went down to see the patient after he passed because I felt an emotional weight I didn't know how to dispel. I went and found the patient's wife because I needed to cry, not necessarily because I wanted to comfort her, or even grieve with her. I had a lot of emotions that I couldn't contain, so I needed a way to act on them.

Still to this day, I feel a lot of emotion behind this experience, I feel heaviness in my chest, tightness in my breathing, my shoulders sagging. I'm not a person that develops emotional bonds easily, so this has been a significant emotional event for me. No one taught me how to have emotional and professional boundaries as a nurse, especially with patients who were "regulars". I also didn't know how to ask for the emotional support that I needed in order to maintain a healthy balance and let go of the intensity of the emotions I was feeling in regards to that patient and that situation.

As a new graduate nurse, I was constantly doubting myself and wondering if there were ways I could have done more to help my patients have a better outcome. As a more experienced nurse now, I've gained more confidence in my skills, but I've also reached a healthier perspective about patients and their health. I realize now that there are many, many factors that are outside my control when it comes to a patient's health. I cannot control their outcome, no matter how much I want to or how much I like them. All I can give is my best, by paying attention to detail, looking them in the eye and giving them dignity as individuals, and advocating for their emotional, spiritual, and physical health. All I can give to myself is the permission to let things go at the end of the day and realize that I am doing the best that I can and that is enough.

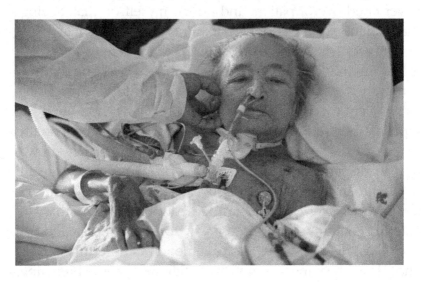

Narrative #2

It was probably within my first year of being off orientation, so less than 2 years of nursing experience when I cared for a 30-something-year-old patient who had a vegetation on one of his heart valves. He was a nervous patient with lots of anxiety who did not like to hear specifics about his care or prognosis because it scared him. This made it difficult for me to feel like I was doing my job to its fullest extent because I felt that I could not explain things properly/fully and discuss with him his feelings on everything going on. I had passed him back and forth with one or two other nurses for at least 2 weeks' worth of shifts. He was a large patient with lots of edema which led to weeping and blistering skin. He required a lot of time calming him down and explaining things without actually explaining details, as he did not like to hear them. I remember it being frustrating and a little confusing of what was the right thing to do and how best to deliver his care.

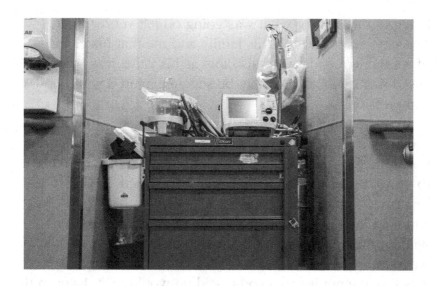

After lots of antibiotics and consults with surgeons, it became clear that he did not have many options; his prognosis was poor and short. His family was more realistic and understood the gravity of the situation, but the patient continued to not want anything explained to him. When I came in for a night shift, I was given report that he had not been looking well all day. His blood pressure was low, he appeared septic, he was lethargic, etc. I remember the off-going RN telling me, "He's probably going to code tonight." I felt scared and stressed and sad for the patient that I had spent a lot of time taking care for. I had only had one patient code before, and I felt very nervous for it to happen again.

I remember that the physicians were very helpful and available, checking in on the patient, which was both a good thing but also a very bad sign; they were very worried about him too. He was a full code.

What was still extra difficult was that the patient did not want to have a discussion about code status, details of his prognosis, or even the fact that everyone was very concerned that he might die that evening. Of course, that is a difficult conversation to have and I can't even imagine to hear, but to have him insist on only talking about positive things and being in the dark of what was going on felt very strange. The physicians had told his family and me that his chances of surviving a code were also low as his valve was so diseased that it would probably be severely injured with chest compressions.

At some point in the shift, the patient asked to be placed on the bed pan. As he was a heavy patient, I had two additional nurses in the room with me to assist. As we rolled him to one side, he started becoming very alarmed, yelling to put him back. Looking at the monitor, I saw that his blood pressure had dipped to about 70/40. We laid him back down without the bed pan as his reaction had happened so quickly we hadn't had time to actually place it. He was nervous, as was I to attempt it again so he said he would wait. Later in the night, he told us he had gone to the bathroom in the bed but was too scared to roll over to get cleaned up. I remember feeling conflicted about this, especially as a new nurse with little experience in judgment of these types of things. I didn't want to leave him soiled, but I also knew the dangers to his life with turning him to clean him with such unstable vital signs. I left him there for a while, which he agreed with and after consulting with several other nurses on the unit, including the charge nurse, we all decided to attempt the turn.

We had five or six nurses there to allow for the quickest, smoothest clean up possible. We rolled him quickly to one side and was able to clean him without anything happening. I felt encouraged by this. We turned him to his right side, which brought his face to my side to clean him up from the other side and he started to panic again. He was yelling "put me down, put me down!" and flailing his arms around. Again, his blood pressure was very low. We immediately laid him back and as I asked if he was ok his head and eyes looked up and to the right and he did not answer me. I shouted his name, staring right into his eyes and I swear I saw the life go out of them. Simultaneously, he became severely bradycardic and his blood pressure went too low, and he coded.

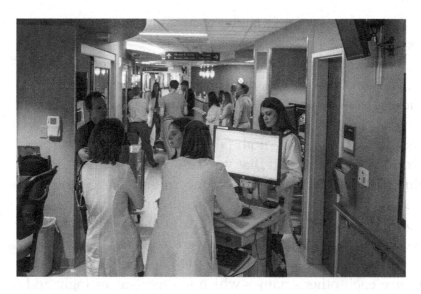

I immediately was able to jump onto his chest with compressions, something I am proud about that I reacted so quickly especially after I had been so nervous and scared. I knew what to do, however, and I did it without hesitating. Because there were so many nurses already in the room with me, everything else went smoothly and quickly too. Someone returned blood from his dialysis machine, someone had the cart and slapped pads on him. The code team arrived not long after. I can't really remember how long we coded him. I know it wasn't that long as his family was there and since they had been educated about his chances, they did not want to prolong anything. It felt like forever though, being such an adrenaline rush. We did everything we could, but we never got him back and it was called. I think what made this so traumatic was that I had taken care of him often, had gotten to know him and he was so young. I was still a new nurse and it was only my second code and the fact that he was still so scared about everything and I could see that in his eyes when he died, made me feel guilty that perhaps it was my fault he died, because we tried to clean him up. The positives were that I was reassured that it wasn't my fault, that it was only a matter of time before that happened and he had to be cleaned up at some point, and I felt very supported throughout the experience.

I remember specifically the physician who ran the majority of the code. He was only an intern as the code team did not arrive immediately and we had worked together on several different shifts. He and I had a good rapport and though he and I were both fairly new to the healthcare world, I felt comforted that we were working together for this patient. I can picture the concern and fear on the physicians face as well, and hear the strain and uncertainty in his voice as he ran the code. But I also remember that because we knew each other and there were so many of my nursing coworkers in the room running the code, we all were able to use each other's names which led to a surprisingly and smoothly run code.

I very clearly remember faces and sights from that experience. I do remember hearing the family members talking to the patient. Some of them were in the room for part of the code and they were almost rooting him on, begging him to come back. Even when family members think they are prepared and understand what is going on and what is happening, in the moment they are still devastated and hoping for a miracle. I think they really realize how traumatic a code is for the patient and for them to witness. And it is traumatic for the healthcare workers of course. Sometimes I think family members need to see some of it for themselves so that they know that everything possible was done for their loved one. Many of the family members, as mentioned, were quite realistic about the situation, so they dealt with it relatively well, but even those who were prepared, I can picture them in the room and in the hallway afterwards, crying and talking to other family members on the phone.

I still struggle to this day with knowing the right thing to say to family members in this situation. I don't think there's actually a right or wrong, set in stone answer to that question, especially because everyone deals with things differently. I want to offer them comfort during a time where that is very difficult to give. I can name most of the people in the room with me and picture where they were in the room. I can see the expressions on their faces. Some looked calm; they had more experience as a nurse and coding patients than I had, plus they hadn't cared for the patient as long as I had.

With the experience I have now, I know that codes still give me an adrenaline rush, but I feel that I have developed the skill, perhaps for lack of a better word, to separate the situation from the patient and family members, in particular if it is not my patient. I think there has to be a certain amount of separation so that we can continue to do our jobs without emotionally burning us out. So some of the nurses in the room I think were able to do that.

I still think of this event when I take care of young patients or people with similar diagnoses. Sometimes when I'm in the room on the unit I also think of him and the whole situation. I remember when the physician mentioned earlier returned to the unit for his third year of internship that I immediately thought of this memory. He mentioned it as well; it impacted both of us and linked us through that situation. When I do think of it though, I always picture the fear in the patient's face, and I find that very disturbing and it causes me to re-experience the feelings and situation as if it is happening to me again.

Physical and Verbal Abuse

One of the most distressing events that happened to me as a nurse occurred when I was working my first overtime shift in the progressive care unit (PCU). This event still causes me distress today.

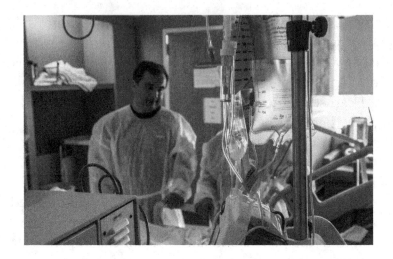

I had an open bed for admission and received a patient from the Emergency Room at about midnight. He was being admitted for alcohol withdrawal, tachycardia and was at high risk for seizure. He was intermittently confused and restless. He was requiring Ativan as needed (PRN) for alcohol withdrawal symptoms about every 2–3 h. The patient also needed IV fluids and a banana bag, but I found that he had pulled both of his peripheral IV (PIV) lines out at about 06:00 right before my shift was ending. I called the physician at this point to let him know that the patient had removed his lines and I did not have access to provide his scheduled medications. I reported to the physician that the patient was refusing to have another PIV inserted and was becoming uncooperative. The physician came to bedside to assess the patient and asked me to re-attempt an IV insertion in order to administer IV Ativan. I asked for the CNA to help me hold his arm steady and pass me supplies when needed. He was calm at the moment, so I was able to insert the IV; however, as I was securing it, the patient became aggressive. He went to swing at me, but the CNA blocked his arm. The patient then spit in my face. I froze, removed the IV that now became half dislodged, and stepped away. The doctor and CNA stood there without saying anything. I couldn't believe what had happened, and I thought to myself that as a nurse I should not have to experience such a thing when I am in a profession to care for others.

I had so many thoughts going through my head. My first thought was anger. I was angry at the patient for treating me like he did. I couldn't believe that someone would spit in the face of someone who was trying to care for them. I realize now that his illness was preventing him from seeing that clearly and that he saw me as the one causing him pain; however, in that moment, all I felt was anger and disbelief. I also felt anger toward the physician for asking me to put a needle in someone who was hostile and combative and then just standing there and not saying anything when the patient spit in my face. He was just going to stand there and watch it all happen? Not even inquire if I was okay? I wondered if this doctor thought that this is what bedside nurses have to endure and that we are just expected to deal with it. I also felt as if I did something wrong. I felt like I should have refused to do an IV under those circumstances or asked for more help to make sure myself and the patient were safe. This caused me to start thinking about the expectations of bedside nurses and how much is asked of us, even if it puts us at risk. After I left the room, I sat down and prepared to give report to the day nurse. I felt frustrated still and almost guilty that I was leaving the nurse with this patient who now did not have an IV line. If only she knew what I went through the just an hour earlier.

The moment this patient spit in my face, I felt so infuriated that I almost checked out for the shift. I had been working so hard to be a good nurse and to help people, and I thought "is this what I get in return?" I have experienced many rewarding moments and met some amazing people throughout my nursing career, but those seemed to go out the window when this happened. I viewed nursing in an overall positive way and felt very hopeful for my nursing career, but this made me question things. I questioned if this is what I wanted to do for the rest of my career, and wasn't sure I could handle many more experiences like that. But looking back, I believe I have experienced many other moments like this. They may not have involved physical abuse, but definitely verbal abuse.

Just a couple of weeks ago, I admitted a patient from the ED (emergency department) and the moment she rolled through the door she rolled her eyes at me, ignored my questions, and said she would have me fired. Here I am, trying to care for you and putting my best foot forward in a positive way and I am immediately treated in a negative way. Someone or something before that time had made this woman extremely upset, and here I was taking the brunt of it. I stood my ground and did not let this woman hurt me emotionally. I told her within the first 10 min, after much verbal abuse, that "I don't know you, and you don't know me, but I am your nurse and here to care for you and help you get better. I will treat you with the utmost respect, and I expect the same from you".

I never thought I would have to endure physical and emotional abuse working as a nurse. I think about these experiences a lot and wonder how long I will be able to continue providing patient care.

Guilt Associated with Bad Care

There was a night shift where I was in charge. I and the rest of my staff had accumulatively maybe about a year of experience, and I was terrified to be the leader of this ship. Being a relief charge nurse with an inexperienced staff was, to me, one of the more horrifying things to experience as a nurse. I remember having thoughts of, "I hope nothing bad happens tonight" and "who can I trust the most with these sick patients?" We didn't get that lucky. One of my nurses admitted a guy named John from the emergency department who sounded like he would be straight forward. My nurse, we will call her Krista, was the one to admit this patient. Krista was a new nurse that I precepted through the new graduate nurse program, so I was familiar with her skill level and also confident that she could handle whatever came up from the emergency department. This man was being transcutaneously paced in the emergency department but now only required a Dopamine drip, and his vital signs were stable. Things were looking up.

The doctor overnight decided that this patient needed a central line. I remember feeling like I needed to check in with the rest of the unit before we placed this line because I knew we would be busy and in the room for a while. As the line was being placed, the patient starts to decondition. There was an increase in oxygen requirement and a rapid need to intubate. I remember having a vivid "oh shit" moment because this patient was going downhill fast and I couldn't figure out why.

What did I miss? I ended up calling a code to get anesthesia there for intubation, and thank god I did because this patient developed pulseless electrical activity (PEA) on the monitor and we had to start resuscitation efforts. CPR was started by Krista and I started meds. The code team showed up and I thought ok, good, we got this. I just needed more hands and more experienced nurses at the bedside to help me. The patient got intubated, which was the only success. Getting IV access on this man was impossible. I asked the code nurse to place an intraosseous cannula and she said no. Wait, what? How do you say no to that? That's your job! Ok I guess I'll do it. The attending running the code asked for a chest tube. I asked for someone to get it but no one knew where it was. Ok I guess I'll get it. Oh, my, are the meds actually going through this intraosseous cannula that I started? Great, it's infiltrating. And this guy isn't getting the lifesaving epinephrine that he needs. I asked the ICU code nurse to start another intraosseous cannula. She said no. Again, what??? How do you say no? Ok I guess I will do it. I was being pulled in every direction because no one knew where anything was. I was the charge nurse and I was supposed to know what to do and to be in a thousand places at once.

Hang on, let me call the chaplain. Wait, did someone send the code labs? What did I miss, how did we get here? This guy was only supposed to need a little dopamine? Did we kill this guy? Blood is everywhere. Vomit is everywhere. Is this really going to be the last way his wife sees him? How awful. It is so loud in here, can other patients hear this? I hope not. Are the other patients ok?? The code lasted forever, but it was like time stood still. I need to use the bathroom but I don't have time!

I remember one day when I was talking to another charge nurse and she told me to always keep my cool because everyone will follow my lead. I thought I was being cool but apparently I wasn't being cool after running my ass of trying to save this guy. What does cool even mean in this moment? Whatever. Can someone call X-ray to get them here? I'll do it.

After a solid hour, we got a pulse back. How? What did we just do to this man? What did I miss? Oh gosh Krista is a mess. The doctor is a mess. That doctor told us that was the single most horrific thing he had ever been through. Great. Glad I could be a part of that. Ugh. This is my fault. Did we really need that central line placed? Did we do this? Why wasn't the shift staffed with more experienced people? Why am I having nightmares still? If only I got that intraosseous cannula placed right the first time. Oh wait, if only someone else helped me place the intraosseous cannula. Gosh I am bitter. This is a mess. I can't wait to come back tomorrow night.

This was a big moment in my career when I questioned my practice as a nurse. Why did I choose this path? There is no other field that holds such responsibility and weight. We are literally taking care of humans. I thought about calling in sick the next shift. I was unsure how I could actually face the family of this patient, my coworkers and the doctors. I felt so heavy. I was so drained. Even pushing the gas pedal down while driving into work felt difficult. I am not in a place to rescue humans from death. I was fearful of the same thing happening again. Feeling under prepared, on edge with every alarm. But I didn't call in. I persevered. How can I call in when we are short staffed? Again. I didn't sleep from the night before. One reason being that I stayed so late after my shift charting the horrific events of the night, explaining the situation to my manager when she came in the morning, and helping clean up the battle scene of that code. I talked with the doctor who ran the code for 30 min before I went home, we held each other and cried. We felt a comradery. This was one of the only people in the world who would understand my feelings. I felt heavy and guilty. But why? We "saved" this man. The other reason I didn't sleep was that I was waking up with nightmares from the code. This surprised me. I have been in so many codes, watched people's souls leave this earth, but why did this one stick so much? All I could see was this man's eyes bulging out of his head, with such intense pressure with the CPR. Blood coming out of everywhere. His mouth, his ears, his chest, his IV sites. Blood was everywhere. How did this happen?? This guy just needed a line. The smell of his emesis was still lofting in my nose. It was sour. It was foul. But moved down this list of problems really quickly compared to not having a heartbeat. The screams of his wife were still curdling my blood. "Please John, please John! NO NO NO!" like a battle cry. I couldn't even think. My thoughts were foggy but yet moving at a million miles a minute. I remember feeling so proud of my staff. Even though they were understaffed and inexperienced, these people were heroes. Everyone stepped up beyond their comfort zone. I felt tearful seeing my cowork-ers the next day. One coworker kissed my check and held me so close, because he was there and felt the same weight I did, he knew how horrific that was. He lived that nightmare. Everyone wanted to hear about the event. I couldn't tell if this was helpful or not. It was nice talking to like-minded people who got the scenario, because my sweet mom sure didn't. She tried to console me when I called her on my way home to tell her that I love her. I was tearful every time I spoke of the event. I was rushed with emotion thinking about those bulg-ing eyes and the hot flush of guilt that I would feel thinking I missed something and how responsible I felt. Although I know we didn't miss anything, I couldn't rationalize this. I couldn't knock the fact that I felt terrible and inept. How can I be a nurse, or even a charge nurse???? The leader on the unit who is supposed to be confident and approachable. And "cool". Right now I was tearful and tired. I needed a vacation, I needed sleep. But John's eyes won't let me.

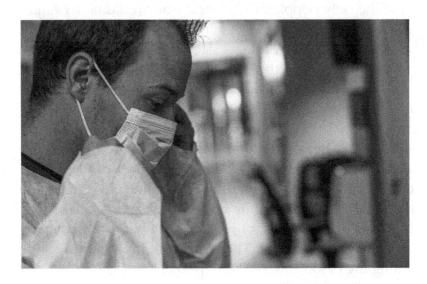

Helping Family Members through Trauma

Narrative #1

A patient was admitted recently to our inpatient unit from a rural outside hospital in Wyoming. The patient was diagnosed with an actively dissecting abdominal aortic aneurysm. She was educated on her options for medical and surgical treatment once she was flown to the hospital for care. Her two options were to undergo surgical intervention to amend her critical condition or to die relatively quickly without surgical intervention. She opted to forgo surgery and completely understood the implications of her decision.

The patient was 58 years old and lived alone with her cat. She appeared to be poorly nourished and unkempt. Most of her family members had been or were currently incarcerated and she did not identify anyone who regularly checked in on her or cared for her in her home. As her medical condition was actively and rapidly declining relatively early on my shift, I asked the resident overseeing her care if she would consider contacting her family member to inform them of these changes. She adamantly declined, stating that she would call the patient's daughter if "something happened". I asked her if that meant she would call the patient's daughter when she died? She avoided my question and carried on with her work. I took it upon myself to contact the patient's daughter and inform her of the changes happening with her mother. I was greeted with the news that she had been released from police custody yesterday and that she had no mode of transportation to make the 6 plus hour drive from her current location. She was hysterical on the telephone and after she passed the phone over to her boyfriend he told me they would try to find a way to make it to the hospital to be with their mother.

Within 3 hours the patient became increasingly more anxious and began complaining of new pain and shortness of breath. She became agonal a few hours later, and by 05:00, she had passed quickly and peacefully. In the last few hours, myself and a few other nurses took time sitting at her bedside and held her hand; providing some final moments of human contact and communicating to her that she wouldn't be alone, even in the most pivotal moments toward her end.

I continued my communication with her daughter throughout the night, as she called and checked in every couple of hours. When she finally passed, the resident asked me if I would call and inform the family, to which I replied that I didn't feel comfortable taking on that responsibility, and I would feel better if an MD performed that roll; a response that was met with resistance from the provider.

It doesn't traumatize or distress me when patients pass whom have chosen that route for the end of their life. It brings me satisfaction and honor to be a part of patient's transitioning in a peaceful and respectful environment. It is part of my role as a nurse; however, in this situation, I felt a certain lack of control that distressed me. I was unable to help her family be with her, and the patient passed much more quickly than she maybe suspected. If she would have known her options before she was transferred out of State, then maybe she could have passed peacefully surrounded by family instead of with complete strangers. I felt unsupported by my physician colleague; pressured to take on additional inappropriate responsibility discussing diagnoses and prognosis and timelines with the family that I was not necessarily trained or equipped to communicate effectively.

I enjoy collaborating with the MD teams very much; however, I felt very unsupported and pressured in this situation. This is not an instance that continues to make me experience residual distress after the fact; however, I do perceive it as a time when I did everything I could do to care for my patient physically and emotionally, and still felt powerless to make the situation positive despite my efforts.

Narrative #2

It was my first and last day with this patient. He was young. I don't remember how old exactly, but I recall thinking he was around my father's age, late forties or early fifties. He was in respiratory failure. For 3 days, his family attempted to wean him off his continuous positive airway pressure (CPAP). For 3 days, they had failed. The patient couldn't tolerate it. His oxygen levels would drop and his breathing grew labored.

The social worker managing his case told me that he had insurance coverage for his hospital stay until the end of the week. It was imperative for the family to agree on goals of care in order to get the patient out of the hospital. The patient was no longer verbal. He couldn't advocate for himself. I'll never forget how his younger brother spoke to him. He told him how much he had always looked up to him. He told him how much he believed in him and that he wanted him to fight this. It broke my heart listening to that. I wondered why no one had sat down with them during the past 3 days and explained to them the chances of him recovering from his respiratory failure.

It seemed like the family was hanging on to false hope. I was so frustrated. I knew in that situation I would want the truth. I remember how exhausting that day was. It was a constant back and forth with the social worker. We talked extensively about what was best for the patient. What the family knew. What they wanted. I remember leaving at the end of the shift thinking I'd never been more tired. The hardest part for me was finally sitting down and telling the family the truth. I explained to the patient's younger brother and his parents that the chances he'd be able to wean off the CPAP successfully were slim. It was the hardest conversation I'd ever had on the job. The family was so appreciative too. They were grateful for my honesty. That made it even more difficult. I held it together in the room. But as soon as I stepped into the hallway, I broke down. I didn't realize the social worker was waiting outside the room for me. She was shocked to see me crying. By that time it was 2:00 or 3:00 in the afternoon, and I hadn't taken even a small break. I'd been going nonstop since 7:00 that morning. I was hungry and exhausted. I couldn't believe I had to be the one to have that hard conversation. I was so frustrated with the physicians. They should have taken the time to explain to the family that the patient was likely never going to get better.

I left my shift that day feeling so defeated. I knew I had done what was best for the patient and his family, but that didn't make me feel much better. The patient transferred to a hospice facility that evening. I knew that was thanks to the care I provided and the tough conversation I was willing to have. But things never should have gotten that far. The family deserved the truth far earlier than when I gave it to them. When I got home, my boyfriend knew something was wrong.

I screamed and cried. I threw things. I know I did what was right. But none of it felt right. Because I was put in an inappropriate situation and forced to suffer the consequences. That was the hardest day of my nursing career.

The feeling I couldn't shake after telling the patient's family he wasn't going to get better was disbelief. It was incredible to me that nurses, doctors, case managers, and social workers had gone in and out of that room for 3 days without bothering to tell the family what they needed to hear. I know it's the doctor's job. But 72h had come and gone and, despite this being my first day with this patient and his family, I was forced to go outside my scope of practice. I was furious. An injustice had been done. And why did I have to pay for that? I provided the care I would have wanted for my own loved one. But that didn't give me any pride or satisfaction. I felt like it was owed to them. Yet no one paid that debt until I was assigned to the patient. I spent only 12 short hours with them, but I did more for my patient and his family in that time than what had been accomplished in the past 3 days. And the worst part? I couldn't even tell you the name of my patient. Or his loved ones. To everyone else, it was just another day on the unit. I know I'm supposed to expound on who was there, but I can't. I can't remember. I want to, but I can't. That's what I find the most infuriating. I just did what was expected of me.

The who, what, when, where, and why didn't matter. Never mind the emotional effect it had on me. It doesn't matter that I cried at work and was humiliated about it. It doesn't matter that I'm sitting here writing this right now. Nobody cares about the aftermath. I did what I had to do because the family had to make a decision before insurance stopped paying for the patient's care. And somehow that was my problem. I wasn't honest with the patient's family because of the money. I told them the patient wasn't getting better because I knew, in that situation that was what I would want to hear. And I hate that I can't remember their names or faces. I only know it was the patient's parents and younger brother, they were the ones whose lives I changed forever. They changed mine.

But on my unit, it was just another day. No one acknowledged my pain or suffering. Just like no one would tell the patient's family the truth they needed to hear. I was mad then, and I'm mad now. It makes me furious to think about how unreasonable nursing can be. It isn't isolated to this incident either. It's every day. The solution to healthcare seems to be asking the nurses to do more things that take away from patient care. Start charting shift notes. Complete your care plans. And don't complain to us if it feels like too much. It's all about patient satisfaction. We couldn't care less about yours. You want to know what I see, hear, and feel? That's what it boils down to every day. Put patient satisfaction before your own needs as a nurse and a human being. Put it above all else. The event I'm writing about, ironically enough, improved the family's satisfaction more than any lie about the patient getting better could have. That's what kills me. Based on this broken healthcare system, I probably shouldn't have told the family the truth about the likelihood of the patient getting better. Because theoretically it would have decreased their satisfaction. But that's the only reason they felt at peace with the situation. Because someone finally told them the truth.

I feel like I don't have an outlet for the anger I have after a tough day on the unit. Part of why I wanted to participate in this writing study was to see if it would help with the challenges I face in nursing. I do try to manage my anger in time spent with my dog. That helps. And over the past year I started working out more regularly. But I don't feel like I'm one of those nurses who can leave job challenges at the workplace. I do feel angry or frustrated about burdens placed on nurses that can be avoided, or aren't necessary in the first place. I think that's where my primary source of anger comes from, the expectations. They're unrealistic, impractical, and a main contributor to burnout in the nursing profession. How I plan to use that in the future? I don't know. Healthcare is a flawed system. It's not something that a single person can change. I just try to do the best for my patients every day. That's what I focus on when I'm at the bedside. And now I'm working on methods of self-care. I continue to try to find healthy emotional outlets. The takeaway from the event that happened, for me, is to never let it happen again. Nursing is about relationships, with the patient, with the family, and with the healthcare team. The best way to foster these relationships is to communicate. A serious lack of communication led to this event in my nursing career, and it's changed how I practice nursing as a result. I strive for transparency as a nurse. And that's a message I plan to share with others.

In conclusion, this chapter has shared powerful personal narratives from nurses. These narratives were labeled as traumatic and experiences that were still causing a level of distress in the nurses' personal and/or professional lives. The use of writing as a resilience intervention to improve cognitive flexibility and cognitive reprocessing will be discussed in Chapters 3 and 5.

Chapter 3

Resilience

As a nurse, you're regularly exposed to stressful and traumatic experiences at work that increase your vulnerability to the harmful and cumulative effects of stress. There are obvious stressors that are inherent to your jobs, which may include situations where you are physically injured or you have to neglect self-care during a shift to take care of your patient assignment. However, it is also important to understand the more nuanced forms of stress and trauma that hold personal meaning and context.

Let's take a look at one common scenario: personal identification with a patient or family. This type of experience might be interpreted as a major trauma in your life that can cause both professional and personal difficulties. What does personally identifying with a patient or family member mean? As an example: you are taking care of a 30-year-old woman who has just delivered her second child. You relate with her because you both are married, are similar in age, and have a three-year-old son at home. After delivery, your patient takes a turn for the worse, develops a bleeding disorder (disseminated intravascular coagulation (DIC)), and is rushed to the intensive care unit for management of her hemorrhaging and resuscitation efforts. The patient's husband is anxiously waiting for news in the waiting room. After 6 h of resuscitation efforts and administering blood and blood products, you and the rest of the medical team are unable to stabilize the patient and she passes away. This is a tragic event for many reasons. Not only have you witnessed the death of a young mother after giving birth to a child, but you are also left grappling with how this has affected you personally. You can't stop thinking about the similarities. You may have ruminating thoughts. What if this was me? What if my husband was left alone to care for our son? Is my son going to be raised without his mother? Or, how does someone so healthy and young die? You may also begin questioning your competence as a nurse or wonder what you could have done differently to prevent this from happening in the first place.

If you are currently a new graduate or a student nurse, and have not been exposed to such an event through clinical rotations or orientation, know that it is inevitable within the career you have chosen. Traumatic or distressing patient experiences may be expected, or they can be completely unpredictable. Regardless, your response to these events will most likely be highly subjective.

You are not a weaker nurse because you care or because a patient experience holds a contextual meaning for you. Quite the opposite. It is important for you to realize the event has had an impact on your life, and to have the ability to process the impact in an appropriate and healthy way. Processing a traumatic or stressful event can be an emotionally nurturing rather than depleting experience. If you are depleted as a nurse, it's hard to imagine that you can show up to work each day or provide an empathetic and/or therapeutic relationship to either your patient or your patient's family. Such emotional depletion also makes it difficult to imagine a long career working at the bedside as a nurse. But processing trauma in a healthy way can allow you to transform the experience and successfully engage the therapeutic use of self in bedside practice.

Processing Stress in the Workplace

As described above, the nuanced and contextual experiences that you bring into nursing may translate into a reaction to a situation that is completely different than your peer's reaction. For some nurses, the stress may be chronic, causing symptoms of anxiety, depression, anger, avoidance, nightmares, and changes in worldview. Left unaddressed, these symptoms can contribute to diagnoses such as burnout syndrome, moral distress, compassion fatigue, posttraumatic stress disorder (PTSD), depression, or anxiety (as discussed in Chapter 1). As a nurse, you may have difficulty sleeping, you may call in to work sick more often and/or, you may use maladaptive coping mechanisms to self-treat these symptoms such as excessive drinking and/or use of prescription or non-prescription medications as a way of easing the pain associated with memories of your experiences. The cascade of symptoms and maladaptive coping may leave you questioning why you became a nurse and whether you chose the right profession.

Nevertheless, many nurses will find a way to meet the challenges associated with stressful patient experiences and continue to enjoy and thrive in the profession for years. It's entirely appropriate for some nurses to have short or acute periods of distress and, after time, translate that stress into an emotionally nurturing experience that allows him/her to continue functioning at the bedside. This is done through the use of healthy coping skills, and in some cases, these skills can help the nurse transcend the experience in a way that promotes growth in the profession.

What is it about these nurses that allows them to bounce back after a poor patient outcome, providing therapeutic empathy to their patients and family members without missing a beat? One theory is increased levels of resilience and the ability to foster resilience within. Resilience is a psychological characteristic that doesn't inoculate you from hardship but allows you to be flexible, bending with adversity and ultimately returning to your baseline functioning or perhaps even a slightly enhanced level of functioning and/or growth.

Defining Resilience

Resilience is defined as the ability to maintain baseline psychological and physical functioning after being exposed to a traumatic or stressful event (Luthar et al., 2000). Resilience has also been recognized as one of the most important factors when assessing adjustment following trauma and is thought to assist in preventing the development of PTSD symptoms (Davidson et al., 2005; Hoge et al., 2007). Factors that promote resilience include individual temperaments, family bonds, and external support systems. Other personal qualities associated with resilience include the ability to engage the support of others, optimism, faith, emotional flexibility, and pursuing personal goals (Davidson et al., 2005; Hoge et al., 2007). These qualities may allow you to cope with stress in an adaptive manner and even thrive in the face of adversity. Most importantly, research has suggested that the personal qualities of resilience, or capacities, as described above, are modifiable and can be taught and learned. Research and inquiry related to resilience has occurred in three waves.

Three Waves of Resilience Inquiry

The first wave identified innate qualities of resilience that allowed people to thrive when faced with internal or external hardship (Richardson, 2002). The innate protective factors were identified as having an easy temperament, being an effective communicator, possessing a sense of personal worth, assertiveness, having above average social skills, having an informal social support network, having the ability to possess close relationships, having an internal locus of control, emotional flexibility, self-confidence, sensitivity to others, trusting others, having a sense of humor, critical thinking and reflection skills, hope, and high expectations (Luthar et al., 2000; Masten, 1994).

Once these innate characteristics were identified, the second wave of inquiry sought to understand how those characteristics could be acquired. Specifically, the second wave looked at internal and external coping skills that could be enriched or modified to serve as protective factors against life stressors (Richardson, 2002). This research included examining biopsychosocial factors of building resilience and how to tolerate stress (Pietrzak et al., 2010; Wu et al., 2013). So how do we teach resilience to others? Resilience can be learned through behavioral change and the development of personal practices or interventions. Resilience interventions can also help strengthen the way we cognitively process situations as well as the thoughts and feelings that assign to those situations (Wu et al., 2013).

Finally, the third wave of resilience inquiry focused on the motivational energy needed to cognitively reframe a life disruption or stressor (Richardson, 2002).

Resilience is applicable to all of life's adversities and any population with uniquely contextual stressors or experiences. Resilience has since been studied by many different groups, including nursing. Nursing has also begun to explore resilience as it relates to moral and ethical challenges experienced in the workplace, which has been coined moral resilience.

Moral Resilience

In 2017, the American Nurses Association (ANA) put together a professional issues steering committee to develop a call to action on moral resilience. Similar to psychological resilience, moral resilience is built in response to adversity, but this is adversity that specifically challenges your moral fabric and serves as an impetus to take action when you are faced with moral and ethical complexities (ANA, 2017).

Group/Institutional Resilience

In addition to individual psychological resilience or moral resilience, researchers suggest the importance of institutional or group resilience. Group level resilience is most influenced by having strong leaders in the work environment (Campbell et al., 2008). It is the leadership behavior that buffers against stressors and promotes mechanisms associated with resilience. Resilient mechanisms include emphasizing work purpose, building and facilitating group cohesion, offering professional support when needed, and empowering peers toward a greater level of control in the work environment (Campbell et al., 2008). By studying whether individual and group characteristics affect resilience in nurses, there is the potential to target recruitment of nurses based on different levels of individual resilience that better fit a particular group. Additionally, this information may help organizational leaders determine where—and to what degree of emphasis—resilience training is needed, and to design systems that increase resilience.

Exploring resilience, moral resilience, and group level resilience as concepts in nursing is relatively new. In the last 10 years, we have seen evidence in the literature about the prevalence of resilience in nurses and also whether resilience interventions are effective at mitigating stress in nursing. Most of the resilience work in nursing seen to date involves the second wave of resilience inquiry and the characteristics of resilience that can be acquired or learned.

Ten Psychological Characteristics of Resilience That Can Be Learned

As discussed earlier in this chapter, certain personal factors and qualities have been identified in highly resilient individuals. Psychologist Dennis Charney and psychiatrist Steven Southwick interviewed survivors of the 9/11 attack on the

World Trade Center, Vietnam prisoners' of war (POWs), Special Forces instructors, and resilient civilians from a variety of environments to identify specific factors and qualities of resilience. Based on these interviews, they were able to identify common themes, leading to ten modifiable resilience factors or coping mechanisms that were effective for dealing with trauma and stress (Southwick & Charney, 2012). The ten coping mechanisms include optimism, developing cognitive flexibility, developing a personal moral compass, altruism, finding resilient role models or mentors, learning how to be adept at facing fear, establishing a social support system, staying physically fit, developing active coping skills, and having a sense of humor (Southwick & Charney, 2012). While this is a valuable foundation, it is not an exhaustive list of resilience factors and there very well may be additional factors that serve as coping mechanisms and buffers to stress.

It isn't necessary to define each of the ten modifiable coping mechanisms because for the most part, they are self-explanatory. However, from a nursing perspective, it is important to address developing cognitive flexibility, establishing a social support system, and developing active coping skills because these characteristics have been found to be important for nurses to cope with their work environment.

Cognitive Flexibility

Cognitive flexibility is a psychological characteristic that involves ability to remain flexible in the way you react to emotion and in the way you think about challenges (Southwick & Charney, 2012). It is the way we deploy coping skills based on the contextual characteristics and variation of situations (Cheng et al., 2012). Using emotional intelligence to guide decision-making in nursing is a good example of cognitive flexibility. Also, managing the emotionally charged atmosphere and emotionally processing direct and indirect traumas through the use of critical reflection, positive reframing, and optimism has been shown to be the effective method incorporated in the workplace by nurses (Mealer et al., 2012b). Below is an example of cognitive flexibility from a nurse with high levels of resilience:

> I don't sit and mull over things. If it was a bad day, I'm sorry it was a bad day and you sort of get on with it. Tomorrow is coming and it will be better.
>
> *(Mealer et al., 2012b, p. 4)*

In contrast, an example of the inflexible or rigid thinking of a nurse who did not have high levels of resilience can be seen as follows:

> It hurts too much to see so much death and so much misery and not be able to do anything about it. I always was a very optimistic upbeat person, but I really feel I have changed since starting to work as a nurse.
>
> *(Mealer et al., 2012b, p. 4)*

These examples are from two nurses who are exposed to both the same type of work environment and patient experiences but derive opposite outlooks based on their level of cognitive flexibility. How can you build the capacity to become flexible to emotions and challenges? Strengthening cognitive flexibility has been explored through a variety of behavioral interventions including exercise (Masley et al., 2009), dance (Coubard et al., 2011), mindfulness (Moore & Malinowski, 2009), and journaling (Pennebaker & Evans, 2014) (see Chapters 4 and 5 for a more detailed description of using mindfulness and journaling to improve your individual resilience).

Social Support

Social support is important for a number of reasons, but I want to describe social support within the context of nursing and how it is possibly linked to building resilience and mitigating stress. My colleagues and I were conducting a pilot resilience training intervention with critical care nurses. Part of the intervention was to attend a 2-day weekend workshop during which we talked about the prevalence of psychological distress in nurses, introduced the nurse participants, and practiced the other components of the intervention. The other components of the intervention involved mindfulness practices, expressive writing, event-triggered cognitive behavioral therapy, and exercise (the results are discussed below). As researchers, we were optimistic that at least one of these practices would resonate with each nurse participant and that after the study concluded, the nurse participant would develop a personal practice outside of the study to continue nurturing his/her individual resilience as a coping strategy for stresses experienced at work. What we learned incidentally through debriefing interviews after the two-day workshop was that the nurse participants felt empowered being in the same room as other nurses who were experiencing the same types of symptoms that they were while at work. The overriding message was that until the workshop, they felt alone and felt like a failure as a nurse. Having difficulty with stress at work is associated with stigma, and therefore, no one talks about it, which leads to isolation within the workplace.

Healthy and secure relationships outside of work are also important. We all know that if we are having problems with our personal relationships, it tends to bleed over into every facet of our lives. Personal social networks and professional social networks are not mutually exclusive, and we need both. A social support network is having that person or persons who you can connect with, communicate with, or receive mentoring from, and someone who can provide you with emotional support when needed. During an interview with a nurse who was struggling with symptoms of anxiety and depression, that nurse shared:

> My assignment was too much for one person and when I appealed for help from the manager, she

continued to berate me over my lack of expertise
and at one point I just said. I really need to be...what
I'm looking for is a mentor that I can feel comfortable going to for help. She just chided me and said I
should really be beyond that point.

(Mealer et al., 2012b, p. 4)

In contrast, being resilient and having the ability to draw upon
the strength of a support network seems to buffer the hardship and emotional struggles that nurses may experience.
After a traumatic event at work, a resilient nurse shared, "It
was really good to sit down and talk about it rather than keep
it into yourself and keep wondering what if" (Mealer et al.,
2012b, p. 4).

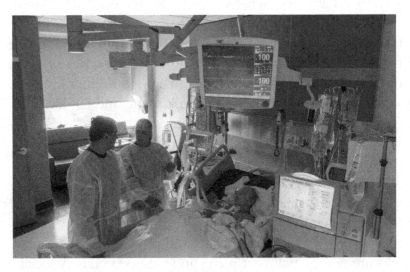

Strengthen your social support network at work. This can
be done formally and institutionally by developing and initi-
ating peer support groups or more informally through peer
gatherings outside of work. The topics of discussion don't
always have to be about work; they could involve a hobby or
other common interests of the group. Eventually, if you get a
group of nurses together, they will talk about work and patient
assignments.

Active Coping Skills

The concept of coping is somewhat abstract but for our purposes encompasses a psychological degree of success or failure in managing a stressful experience. The goal of active coping skills is to reduce subjective levels of stress or distress by either modifying your environment to interact with a stressor or removing the stressor altogether. Similar to resilience, the concept of coping can be an innate personality trait or a capacity that changes over time and based on the situation being encountered. Every individual has both internal and external approaches to coping and most likely has acquired a group of strategies that have been successful in the past. If a strategy or skill has been used successfully in the past, you are more likely to draw upon that skill for a similar situation.

It is also important to classify coping skills as healthy or unhealthy. You can successfully manage a stressful experience at work, but the consequence may be deleterious to your physical and emotional health. As a nurse, physical health may include exercise, nutrition, and sleep habits, while emotional health may include remembering the positive experiences you've had at work and the ability to leave traumatic or emotional stress at work instead of carrying it home to your personal life.

Nurses with unhealthy coping skills have described using substances, such as alcohol, daily as an adjunct for sleep or as a means to calm their troubling thoughts about patient encounters that were traumatic or associated with poor outcomes. In contrast, nurses using healthy coping skills describe both internal and external strategies when dealing with work-related stress. For example, one nurse shared this internal coping strategy: "Before I go to work, I clear my mind for the day. I actually say a prayer to be a vessel to be used that day. It's my daily ritual." Another nurse shared this external coping strategy: "I exercise because I think that one of the things about nursing...it is a giving profession and I think that you have to do things so that you don't...so that you have that to give the next day."

As mentioned earlier, acquiring or learning resilient characteristics allows you to experience an adverse situation while also accessing strengths and positive coping mechanisms to grow through the experience. We've described internal and external coping skills as well as healthy and unhealthy coping skills, but ultimately, it is practicing and nurturing these skills when you are caring for patients that will help develop active coping skills as a resilience characteristic. Building resilience through the use of active coping skills, a supportive social network, and cognitive flexibility is entirely within your means, but it will take time and sustained effort.

Measuring Resilience

To understand resilience levels in nursing, we first need to understand how resilience is measured and how to interpret the measurement scores. Resilience is not an all or none concept, and there are varying degrees with higher scores indicating higher levels of resilience. There are several instruments that have been developed to measure resilience, but the instrument with the most robust psychometric testing that has been more commonly used in healthcare professionals is the Connor Davidson Resilience Scale (CD-RISC).

Connor Davidson Resilience Scale

The CD-RISC is a 25-item self-report scale with scores ranging from 0 to 100. Higher scores indicate greater levels of resilience (Mealer et al., 2012a). The conceptual factors that make up the content of the CD-RISC include personal competence; having high standards and tenacity; trusting your instincts; the ability to tolerate the negatives and gain strength from stress; being accepting of change; and having good secure relationships, control, and spirituality. When the scale was originally developed, it was tested in a variety of populations including the general population, primary care setting, psychiatric inpatient, and clinical trials population. In these populations, there was good validity, internal consistency, and test–retest reliability reported. The intent of this scale was to provide a valid and reliable measure of resilience and establish references values for being resilient or non-resilient in both the general population and clinic populations (Connor & Davidson, 2003).

Resilience in Nursing

Our research team sought to determine the prevalence of resilience in ICU nurses and whether the presence of resilience was associated with improved psychological functioning and fewer symptoms of distress. To do this, we sent out a survey to a national sample of critical care nurses who were members of the American Association of Critical Care Nurses (AACN). In addition to the CD-RISC to measure resilience, the survey included validated questionnaires on symptoms of anxiety, depression, burnout syndrome, and PTSD.

Over 700 nurses responded and of those who responded, 22% were considered to be highly resilient based on their CD-RISC score. The highly resilient nurses were less likely to have symptoms of PTSD (8% vs. 25%, $p < 0.001$) anxiety (8% vs. 21%, $p = 0.003$) or depression (2% vs. 14%, $p < 0.001$). Burnout syndrome symptoms in the dimensions of emotional exhaustion, depersonalization, and a reduced sense of personal accomplishment were also significantly lower in nurses who were highly resilient.

As nurses, we know that we can sometimes take our work home with us. In this national survey, we asked nurses if their work effected their functioning outside of the hospital. Highly

resilient nurses were less likely to report problems with friend-
ships (5% vs. 21%, $p < 0.001$), relationships with their family
(7% vs. 21%, $p < 0.001$), engaging in fun or leisurely activities
(9% vs. 22%, $p = 0.003$), general satisfaction with life (8% vs.
27%, $p < 0.001$), and their overall level of functioning (5% vs.
22%, $p < 0.001$) (Mealer et al., 2012a).

Obviously, the above results were quite encouraging, and
we wanted to understand what highly resilient nurses were
doing to adequately cope with their work as a bedside nurse.
Through qualitative interviews, we were able to identify specific resilience characteristics that have guided the development of interventions to help build resilience and potentially
mitigate distress in nurses.

The first resilience pilot study that we conducted looked
at the feasibility and acceptability of a multimodal resilience
intervention over 12 weeks. The intervention included a
writing intervention, event-triggered cognitive behavioral coun-
seling sessions, mindfulness techniques, and a protocolized
exercise regimen.

Writing

The writing sessions were led by experts who were trained
in motivational interviewing and resilience. Nurse participants were given weekly writing prompts and were asked to
write for 30 min each week. The writing prompts involved
work-related topics and the feedback provided by our experts
encouraged resilience-building practices.

Event-Triggered Counseling Sessions

A licensed counselor trained in traumatic stress delivered
therapy sessions with the nurse participants if, during a work
shift, the nurse experienced a patient's death, participated in

end-of-life family discussions, performed cardiopulmonary resuscitation on a patient, participated in futile care with a terminal patient, cared for a patient with traumatic injuries, and/or cared for a patient with massive bleeding. These therapy sessions were aimed at challenging negative thoughts and promoting resilience through cognitive flexibility and restructuring. We chose event-triggered sessions in an attempt to relieve the stigma associated with seeking help for work-related distress.

Mindfulness Practices

The mindfulness practices were introduced at a workshop by a mindfulness-based stress reduction (MBSR) expert. The body scan and sitting meditation were the techniques that were demonstrated and practiced in person. A guided CD of these techniques was provided to participants for home practice. Each nurse participant was asked to practice for 15 min, three times per week.

Aerobic Exercise

The exercise protocol consisted of aerobic activities that could include using the treadmill, elliptical machine, stair climber, stationary bicycle, or rowing machine at our institution's wellness center. The study budget covered the cost of the memberships. Each nurse participant was asked to exercise 30–45 min at least three times per week.

The multimodal intervention was successfully implemented with adherence to each component that ranged from 66% to 100%. There were no dropouts from the study, and each component received high satisfaction scores. Although not sufficiently powered to determine the effectiveness of the intervention at mitigating symptoms of psychological distress, there were significant increases in resilience scores and significant decreases in symptoms of depression and PTSD in pre- and post-participation scores. This was the first intervention in ICU nurses that adopted a multifaceted approach to teaching resilience (Mealer et al., 2014).

In conclusion, as living organisms, we are always striving to reach homeostasis, or a return to our previous state of functioning. When faced with adversity, depending on your ability to access protective and resilient characteristics, you may reintegrate resiliently, reintegrate back to homeostasis, reintegrate with loss, or reintegrate with dysfunction. We know that possessing resilient traits is advantageous, but can resilience interventions successfully reduce symptoms of distress in nurses and improve objective resilience scores? Since this original pilot study, there have been several other resilience intervention studies tested in nursing with a particular highlight on mindfulness and written exposure therapy. Chapters 4 and 5 will provide more detail in the use of mindfulness and writing to improve resilience in nursing.

References

American Nurses Association (2017). Exploring moral resilience toward a culture of ethical practice: a call to action report. Retrieved from: www.nursingworld.org/~4907b6/globalassets/docs/ana/ana-call-to-action--exploring-moral-resilience-final.pdf.

Campbell, D., Campbell, K. & Ness, J.W. (2008). Resilience through leadership. In B.J. Lukey & V. Tepe (Eds.). *Biobehavioral Resilience to Stress* (pp. 57–88). New York: CRC Press.

Cheng, C., Kogan, A. & Chio, J. (2012). The effectiveness of a new, coping flexibility intervention as compared with a cognitive-behavioral intervention in managing work stress. *Work & Stress*, 3, 272–288.

Connor, K.M. & Davidson, J.R. (2003). Development of a new resilience scale: The Connor-Davidson Resilience Scale (CD-RISC). *Depression and Anxiety*, 18, 76–82.

Coubard, O.A., Duretz, S., Lefebvre, V., Lapalus, P. & Ferrufino, L. (2011). Practice of contemporary dance improves cognitive flexibility in aging. *Frontiers in Aging Neuroscience*, 3, 1–12.

Davidson, J.R., Payne, V.M., Connor, K.M., Foa, E.B., Rothbaum, B.O., Hertzberg, M.A. & Weisler, R.H. (2005). Trauma, resilience and saliostasis: Effects of treatment in post-traumatic stress disorder. *International Clinical Psychopharmacology*, 20, 43–48.

Hoge, E.A., Austin, E.D. & Pollack, M.H. (2007). Resilience: Research evidence and conceptual `considerations for posttraumatic stress disorder. *Depression and Anxiety*, 24, 139–152.

Luthar, S., Cicchetti, D. & Becker, B. (2000). The construct of resilience: A critical evaluation and guidelines for future work. Child Development, 71, 543–562.

Masley, S., Roetzheim, R. & Gualtieri, T. (2009). Aerobic exercise enhances cognitive flexibility. *Journal of Clinical Psychology in Medical Settings*, 16, 186–193.

Masten, A.S. (1994). Resilience in individual development: Successful adaptation despite risk and adversity. In M.C. Wang & E.W. Gordon (Eds.), *Educational Resilience in Inner-City America: Challenges and Prospects* (3–25). Hillsdale, NJ: Erlbaum.

Mealer, M., Jones, J., Newman, J., McFann, K., Rothbaum, B. & Moss, M. (2012a). The presence of resilience is associated with a healthier psychological profile in intensive care unit (ICU) nurses: Results of a national survey. *International Journal of Nursing Studies*, 49, 292–299.

Mealer, M., Jones, J. & Moss, M. (2012b). A qualitative study of resilience and posttraumatic stress disorder in United States ICU nurses. *Intensive Care Medicine*, 38, 1445–1451.

Mealer, M., Conrad, D., Evans, J., Jooste, K., Solyntjes, J., Rothbaum, B. & Moss, M. (2014). Feasibility and acceptability of a resilience training program for intensive care unit nurses. *American Journal of Critical Care*, 23, 97–105.

Moore, A. & Malinowski, P. (2009). Meditation, mindfulness and cognitive flexibility. *Consciousness and Cognition*, 18, 176–186.

Pennebaker, J. & Evans, J. (2014). *Expressive Writing: Words that Heal.* Enumclaw, WA: Idyll Arbor.

Pietrzak, R.H., Johnson, D.C., Goldstein, M.B., Malley, J.C., Rivers, A.J., Morgan, C.A. & Southwick, S.M. (2010). Psychosocial buffers of traumatic stress, depressive symptoms, and psychosocial difficulties in veterans of Operations Enduring Freedom: The role of resilience, unit support and postdeployment social support. *Journal of Affective Disorders*, 120, 188–192.

Richardson, G.E. (2002). The metatheory of resilience and resiliency. *Journal of Clinical Psychology*, 58, 307–321.

Southwick, S. & Charney, D. (2012). *Resilience: The Science of Mastering Life's Greatest Challenges*. Cambridge: Cambridge University Press.

Wu, G., Feder, A., Cohen, H., Kim, J.J., Calderon, S., Charney, D.S. & Mathe, A.A. (2013). Understanding resilience. *Frontiers in Behavioral Neuroscience*, 7, 1–15.

Chapter 4

Mindfulness Practices

Background

Mindfulness is a practice that has been around for thousands of years and embraced in both religious and non-religious settings by many of the Asian countries. Kabat-Zinn (2013) has defined mindfulness as "tuning in to each moment in an effort to remain awake and aware from one moment to the next" (p. 6). From a Buddhist perspective, mindfulness is the art of stopping, and with cultivation will help temper ruminative thinking, forgetfulness, strong emotions, and habit energies that control us (Nhat-Hanh, 2015). Habit energies are similar to automatic thoughts or actions, habituated by family and societal belief systems that can be highly imbued with strong emotions and are typically outside of our volitional control. We can stop these habit energies by practicing mindfulness. Nhat-Hanh (2015) describes mindfulness as "the energy that allows us to recognize our habit energy and prevent it from dominating us" (p. 25).

Within the last several decades, Western psychology has taken the traditional mindfulness practices of Eastern philosophy and combined those practices with contemporary psychology to improve wellbeing and health outcomes. With this effort, we have also seen standardized mindfulness practices, which promotes scientific rigor as we try to determine if mindfulness is an effective treatment for a variety of different health conditions. The two main mindfulness-based interventions (MBIs) are mindfulness-based stress reduction (MBSR) and mindfulness-based cognitive therapy (MBCT).

MBSR and MBCT are very similar. They both include eight-weekly two-hour in-person sessions plus a one-day retreat. These are group-based therapies of formal and informal mindfulness practices. The mindfulness practices are introduced by an instructor, practiced during sessions, and it is expected that participants will devote time for home practice. The mindfulness interventions include mindfulness of the breath, thoughts, bodily sensations, emotions, sounds, and everyday activities. Following in-session mindfulness practice, there is an instructor-guided inquiry into the practice, which is a method used by instructors to help the participant identify thoughts, feelings, and emotions that contribute to automated patterns or habits that can contribute to negative moods. The process of inquiry fosters a mindful way of relating to experiences with self-compassion and a non-judgmental awareness of the present moment.

Although very similar, two differences that are worth noting between standardized MBSR and MBCT are group membership and the role of cognitive therapy. As the name implies, MBCT combines the Eastern philosophy techniques of MBSR with cognitive therapy and specifically uses a technique known as decentering. Decentering is the ability to see your thoughts from a wider perspective. Imagine being able to press a pause button whenever you have a strong emotion or are put in a stressful situation. The pause button, or decentering, allows you to separate yourself from the experience, which ultimately changes the nature of the experience (Bernstein et al., 2015). Gaining insight into mood through the technique of decentering further validates that our beliefs and emotions are used to model and assign meaning to thoughts (i.e., positive or negative). Because of this, the didactic portion of MBCT uses scenarios with common symptoms, thoughts, and emotions of a particular disorder. Traditionally, MBCT was developed to prevent depression relapse but has since been modified for anxiety disorders, posttraumatic stress disorder (PTSD), postpartum depression, substance use disorders, and burnout syndrome. Therefore, unlike MBSR, the eight-week MBCT classes have a homogenous group of participants.

Mindfulness is being able to truly experience the present moment, and although we can't change the essence of nursing or caring for sick patients, sometimes critically and traumatically ill, we can change our relationship with these stressful experiences. However, there isn't robust evidence to support mindfulness practices for the treatment of burnout syndrome, and these classes alone may not be enough for long-term relief of symptoms related to chronic work stressors. For the individual nurse, it will take continued work and practice to develop a sustainable personal mindfulness practice.

Mindfulness and Use in Healthcare

We know from evidence in the literature that mindfulness practices have been used quite effectively for medical treatment in a variety of patient populations including those with chronic pain, breast cancer recovery, and depression (Carlson et al., 2015; Dimidjian & Goodman, 2014; Garland et al., 2015; Teasdale et al., 1995). But what about healthcare providers and, in particular, what about nurses?

In a recent meta-analysis of mindfulness in healthcare providers, results suggest that MBIs significantly decreased stress levels in healthcare providers. This meta-analysis included studies that involved the evaluation of an MBI intervention, healthcare professionals, and a pre- and post-outcome measure of stress. The MBIs involved traditional MBSR, modified versions of MBSR, mindfulness-based cognitive attitude training, and telephonic MBSR. Out of 472 potential studies that were identified from MEDLINE, PsychINFO, CDINAHL, and BNI, only nine studies remained eligible for the analysis. The results identified a medium effect side ($r = 0.342$) (CI = 0.202–0.468) and a combined probability of $p < 0.00002$ (Burton et al., 2017).

Our group has started to look at mindfulness and how MBIs may help improve symptoms of stress in the workplace. There is still the need for large randomized controlled trials that are powered to determine the effectiveness of MBIs for mitigating stress and improving resilience, but the pilot studies to date have looked quite promising. In 2014, we conducted a multimodal pilot study that recruited critical care nurses into a 12-week randomized controlled clinical trial. Nurses were included if they worked at least 20h per week in the intensive care unit (ICU) and if they scored ≤82 on the CD-RISC, which indicated lower levels of resilience. The multimodal intervention included exercise, event-triggered cognitive behavioral therapy (CBT), expressive writing, and mindfulness practices.

The mindfulness practices included the body scan, sitting meditation, and walking meditation, which were introduced and practiced over a two-day weekend educational workshop. After the two-day workshop concluded, participants were provided a guided CD that could be used for home practice, and home practice was expected to occur at least three times a week for 15min. After the 12-week intervention, results indicated that the nurses engaged in these MBIs on average of 65min per week, there were significant reductions in symptoms of depression and symptoms of PTSD, and there were significant improvements in resilience scores. Further research is needed since this was primarily a feasibility and acceptability study, and the MBIs were only a piece of a multimodal intervention. Nonetheless, these are promising results (Mealer et al., 2014).

More recently, we have started to look at MBCT and how this traditional eight-week treatment may be adapted and used with critical care nurses to reduce burnout syndrome and improve resilience. However, working 12-h shifts sometimes 3 or 4 days in a row makes it difficult to find a consistent day and time that would work for eight-weekly two-hour group classes. To better understand the feasibility of an MBCT resilience intervention for nurses, we conducted focus groups with nurses who were members of the American Association of Critical Care Nurses (AACN). We were specifically interested in MBCT adaptation data related to the preferred timing of the MBCT sessions, preferred format (face-to-face or online), qualifications of the MBCT instructor, and the feasibility of daily homework and the amount of homework/time commitment per day.

The four domains that were identified through these interviews included barriers to adherence, incentives for adherence, preferred qualifications of instructors, and the didactic content that would address ICU-specific triggers of burnout syndrome and psychological distress. Barriers to adherence, as expected, included the length of the sessions were thought to be too long; there were potential childcare concerns, difficulty attending if after a shift or after consecutive 12-h shifts, concerns about work–home life balance and the length of time practicing at home. It was felt that participating in an MBCT resilience intervention could be incentivized by providing a stipend and/or salary coverage for attendance, providing a hybrid session of online/face-to-face sessions, including mindfulness practices that could be completed at work and using alternative methods to provide didactic content such as podcasts that could be listed to while driving to work or multitasking when home. The focus group participants also felt that the instructor should have expertise in the delivery of MBCT but should also have nursing experience. As mentioned previously in this chapter, MBCT uses decentering as a cognitive method to address negative mood and ultimately change our relationship with negative thoughts and emotions. Therefore, understanding the nurse's perspective and ICU-specific triggers of distress that could be folded into didactic content was extremely valuable. The triggers ranged from supply carts not being restocked to emotional injuries and guilt associated with poor care (Mealer et al., 2017). The results of these qualitative interviews have been used to modify the traditional MBCT sessions, and we are currently in the process of conducting a feasibility and acceptability clinical trial in nurses as an intervention to build resilience and reduce workplace distress.

Mindfulness has been described in nursing as an important component of self-regulation in response to distress and adversity and a strategy to promote moral resilience (ANA, 2017). Furthermore, nurses, who practice mindfulness interventions as a technique to promote positive coping during stress, are found to be more effective in increasing organizational as well as individual resilience (Foureur et al., 2013).

This all sounds great, but ultimately, we do not have the evidence to definitively state that mindfulness is beneficial for nurses who are experiencing distress as a result of the work environment. Research takes time, and more importantly, randomized controlled trials cost money. Unfortunately, there are scarce financial resources to support this line of research. Below, I will provide the rationale and instructions for a few mindfulness interventions that can be practiced at home. This will include the sitting meditation, the 3-min breathing space exercise, and the body scan meditation. Make a commitment to yourself to develop your own personal mindfulness practice and see if you notice improvements in your symptoms of distress and burnout.

Sitting Meditation

Sitting meditation has been around for centuries and meant to be a simplistic practice but not necessarily an easy practice. Simplistic because we sit every day, and the only instructions are awareness of the breath and awareness of "being" instead of "doing." Herein lies the difficulty, particularly for nurses who are constantly in the "doing-mode" and for whom there are potentially life or death consequences for not doing.

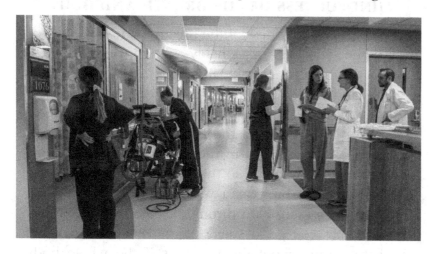

It is difficult to not let the mind wander to tasks that you should be doing, things that you forgot to do or what you plan on doing in the future. Some people think that they are not doing a good job or practicing incorrectly because their mind wanders during sitting meditation practices. To the contrary, this is expected. Even individuals who have been meditating for years will have episodes where their mind wanders but merely acknowledging that the mind has wandered and bringing awareness back to the breath is all that is expected.

To begin sitting meditation, find a comfortable place to sit and a place that you will not be interrupted. You can sit on the floor or on a chair, whichever is most comfortable. Sit with a dignified, erect, and alert posture. Individuals that have never practiced mindfulness in the past sometimes think that they are supposed to feel calm and relaxed after a session of mindfulness or sitting meditation. This can sometimes be true but that isn't the point of the exercise. The point is to be present in the moment, whether there is comfort or discomfort and to recognize that your thoughts and emotions are temporarily passing through and dependent on context. Box 4.1 provides detailed instructions on performing sitting meditation.

**BOX 4.1: SITTING MEDITATION:
MINDFULNESS OF THE BREATH AND BODY**

1. Practice mindfulness of the breath for 10–15 min.
2. When you feel reasonably settled on awareness of the breath, intentionally allow the awareness to expand around the breath to include, as well, a sense of physical sensations throughout the whole body. While still aware, in the background, of the movements of the breath in the lower abdomen, change your primary focus, so that you become aware of a sense of the body as a whole and of the changing patterns of sensation throughout the body. You may find that you get a sense of the movements of the breath throughout the body, as if the whole body were breathing.
3. If you choose, together with this wider sense of the body as a whole, and of the breath moving to and from, include awareness of the more local, particular patterns of physical sensations that arise where the body makes contact with the floor, chair, cushion, or stool—the sensations of touch, pressure, or contact of the feet or knees with the floor; the buttocks with which whatever supports them; and the hands where they rest on the thighs or on each other. As best you can, hold all these sensations, together with the sense of the breath and of the body as a whole, in a wider space of awareness of physical sensations.
4. The mind will wander repeatedly away from the breath and body sensations—this is natural, to be expected, and in no way a mistake or a failure. Whenever you notice that your awareness has drifted away from sensations in the body, you might want to congratulate yourself; you have "woken up." Gently note where your mind was ("thinking"), and kindly focus your

attention back to your breathing and to a sense of your body as a whole.

5. As best you can, keep things simple, gently attending to the actuality of sensations throughout your body from one moment to the next.

6. As you sit, some sensations may be particularly intense, such as pains in the back, knees, or shoulders, and you may find that awareness is repeatedly drawn to these sensations, and away from your intended focus on the breath or body as a whole. You may want to use these times to experiment with choosing intentionally either to shift posture, or to remain still and bring the focus of awareness into the region of intensity. If you choose to remain still, then, as best you can, explore with gentle and wise attention the detailed pattern of sensations here: What, precisely, do the sensations feel like? Where exactly are they? Do they vary over time or from one part of the region of intensity to another? Not so much thinking about them, as just feeling them. You may want to use the breath as a vehicle to carry awareness into such regions of intensity, "breathing in" to them, just as in the body scan. Breathe out from those sensations, softening and opening with the outbreath.

7. Whenever you find yourself "carried away" from awareness in the moment of the intensity of physical sensations, or in any other way, remind yourself that you can always reconnect with the here and now by refocusing awareness on the movements of the breath or on a sense of the body as a whole. Once you have gathered yourself in this way, allow the awareness to expand once more, so it includes a sense of sensations throughout the body.

8. And now for the last few moments of this sitting, bringing your attention back to focus on your breathing

in the abdomen. Tuning in to any and all sensations on this inbreath and this outbreath. And as you sit here and as you breathe, allowing yourself to cultivate this sense of moment-to-moment awareness, and remembering that the breath is available to you at any moment of your day, to allow you to feel grounded, to give a sense of balance and an awareness of accepting yourself as you are in each moment.

Three-Minute Breathing Space Exercise

Sitting meditation may be more appropriate for home practice than when you are in the middle of a busy shift in the hospital or clinic setting. Finding shorter exercises that can be used to diffuse stressful or traumatic situations experienced at work, or an exercise that can be used as a simple reset to nourish the mind during a busy shift, may be important for mitigating workplace stress but also in developing a sustainable personal mindfulness practice.

As a nurse, sometimes you won't have time to take a lunch/ dinner break or even use the restroom, so it would be difficult to practice a mindfulness exercise that lasted longer than 3 min. Find the opportunities to make this work for your schedule. I can think of several occasions where a 3-min mindfulness break would be feasible, such as when you take a bathroom break; when you are on the phone holding to speak with a physician or other ancillary department staff; when you have traveled to MRI or the CT scanner for a procedure; waiting to report off to the oncoming shift; when you are walking from the parking lot before or after a shift; and/or during a scheduled meal break (knowing that this may or may not happen).

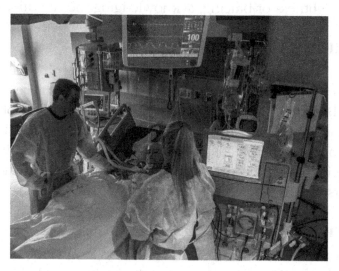

Box 4.2 provides detailed instructions on the 3-min breathing space exercise.

BOX 4.2: THE THREE-MINUTE BREATHING SPACE: INSTRUCTIONS

STEP 1: BECOMING AWARE

Become more aware of how things are in this moment by deliberately adopting an erect and dignified posture, whether sitting or standing. If possible, close your eyes. Then, bringing your awareness to your inner experience and acknowledging it, ask "What is my experience *right now?*"

■ What *THOUGHTS* are going through your mind? As best you can, acknowledge thoughts as mental events, perhaps putting them into words.
■ What *FEELINGS* are here? Turn toward any sense of discomfort or unpleasant feelings, acknowledging them.

■ What *BODY SENSATIONS* are here right now? Perhaps quickly scan the body to pick up any sensations of tightness or bracing, acknowledging the sensations.

STEP 2: GATHERING

Then, redirect your attention to focus on the physical sensations of the breathing itself. Move in close to the sense of the breath in the abdomen…feeling the sensations of the abdomen wall expanding as the breath comes in…and falling back as the breath goes out. Follow the breath all the way in and all the way out, using the breathing to anchor yourself into the present.

STEP 3: EXPANDING

Now expand the field of your awareness around the breathing so that it includes a sense of the body as a whole, your posture, and facial expression.

If you become aware of any sensations or discomfort, tension, or resistance, take your awareness there by breathing into them on the inbreath. Then, breathe out from those sensations, softening and opening with the outbreath.

As best you can, bring this expanded awareness to the next moments of your day.

Body Scan Meditation

The body scan meditation is usually the first practice and the longest practice that is learned in an MBSR or MBCT class. The body scan is a systematic approach to fostering awareness of breath, and it is the underpinning for many of the formal mindfulness interventions that may be participated in by an individual. As the name implies, the body scan is a detailed awareness of the body from the toes to the top of the head. This is important because thoughts and emotions are often manifested in the body such as anxiety causing tension in the shoulders or tightness in the chest. A better sense of how the body feels provides valuable insight to identify negative ways of feeling and thinking (Teasdale et al., 1995).

The body scan is practiced while lying down. Since this is a 45-min exercise, you should find a time to complete the body scan when you feel rested and not overly sleepy. Similar to sitting meditation, the body scan is not meant to be relaxing, although it may be. If you find that you are falling asleep when you practice the body scan, choose a different time of day when you feel fully awake and alert or attempt the scan with your eyes open instead of closed. This is an exercise of awareness and with practice, an exercise of "'falling awake', of learning how to relax into awareness" (Teasdale et al., 1995, p. 155). Box 4.3 provides detailed instructions on performing the body scan.

BOX 4.3: THE BODY SCAN MEDITATION

1. Lie down on your back in a comfortable place, such as on a foam mat or pad on the floor or on your bed. Keep in mind from the very beginning that in this lying-down practice, the intention is to "fall awake" rather than fall asleep. Make sure that you will be warm enough. You might want to cover yourself with a blanket or do it in a sleeping bag if the room is cold.
2. Allow your eyes to gently close. But if and when you find any drowsiness creeping in, feel free to open your eyes and continue with them open.
3. Gently let your attention settle on your abdomen, feeling the rise and falling of your belly with each inbreath

and each outbreath, in other words "riding the waves" of your own breathing with full awareness for the full duration of each inbreath and the full duration of each outbreath.

4. Take a few moments to feel your body as a whole, from head to toe; the "envelope" of your skin; the sensations associated with touch in the places you are in contact with the floor or the bed.

5. Bring your attention to the toes of the left foot. As you direct your attention to them, see if you can direct or channel your breathing to them as well, so that it feels as if you are breathing in to your toes and out from your toes. It may take a while for you to get the hang of this so that it doesn't feel effortful or contrived. It may help to imagine your breath traveling down the body from your nose into the lungs and continuing through the torso and down the left leg all the way to the toes, and then back again and out through your nose. Actually, the breath does take this and every other route in the body, through the bloodstream.

6. Allow yourself to feel any and all sensations from your toes, perhaps distinguishing between them and watching the flux of sensations in this region. If you don't feel anything at the moment, that is fine too. Just allow yourself to feel "not feeling anything."

7. When you are ready to leave the toes and move on, take a deeper, more intentional breath in all the way down to the toes, and, on the outbreath, allow them to "dissolve" in your mind's eye. Stay with your breathing for a few breaths at least, and then move on in turn to the sole of the foot, the heel, the top of the foot, and then the ankle, continuing to breathe in to and out from each region as you observe the sensations

that you are experiencing, and then letting go of that region and moving on.

8. As with the sitting meditation exercise, bring your mind back to the breath and to the region you are focusing on each time you notice that your attention has wandered off, after first taking note of what carried you away in the first place or what is on your mind when you realize it has wandered away from the focus of the body.

9. In this way, continue moving slowly up your left leg and through the rest of your body as you maintain the focus on the breath and on the sensations within the individual regions as you come to them, breathe with them, and let go of them.

10. Practice the body scan at least once a day.

11. Remember that the body scan is the first formal mindfulness practice introduced in MBSR and it is done for 45 min a day, 6 days a week, for at least 2 weeks straight in the beginning of training. So when you are ready, that would be a good strategy for undertaking the next steps in your own developing meditation practice, especially if you want to follow the full curriculum of MBSR and give it and yourself a fair chance.

12. If you have trouble staying awake, try doing the body scan with your eyes open, as noted in step 2 above.

13. The most important point is to get down on the floor and practice. How much or for how long is not as important as that you make the time for it at all, every day if possible.

Excerpt(s) from FULL CATASTROPHE LIVING by Jon Kabat-Zinn, copyright © 1990 by Jon Kabat-Zinn. Used by permission of Dell Publishing, an imprint of Random House, a division of Penguin Random House LLC. All rights reserved.

Other Treatments Involving Mindfulness

Mindfulness is a behavioral therapy and thus requires practice and, as discussed previously, involves an individual commitment to developing a personal practice. Behavior therapy can be divided into three generations including traditional behavior therapy, CBT, and most recently contextual approaches or the "third generation" of behavior and cognitive therapy, which includes acceptance and commitment therapy (ACT) and dialectical behavior therapy (DBT).

Acceptance and Commitment Therapy

ACT is an evidence-based treatment that uses cognitive defusion and mindfulness to increase behavioral flexibility. It is a non-judgmental acceptance and embracing of the experience as it is in the present moment. ACT is considered a third-wave psychotherapy and is used for a variety of symptoms, including anxiety and depression (Hayes, 2004).

ACT involves six core processes:

- *Acceptance* is the first core process, and it is taught as an alternative to avoiding experiences that may cause distress.
- Second is *cognitive defusion* or the attempt to change the relationship one has with thoughts by adding contextual experiences to gradually decrease the attachment or factual beliefs assigned to a thought. This is similar to the decentering technique of MBCT described earlier in the chapter.
- The third process is "*being present.*" ACT fosters non-judgmental relationships with thoughts, emotions, and environmental events and "being present" through the use of mindfulness practices.
- *The self as concept* is the fourth core process and is described as a context for verbal knowing, not the actual

content of the knowing. This process is promoted in ACT through experiential processes, metaphors, and mindfulness exercises.

■ ACT uses exercises to promote *values* by helping individuals choose directions as it relates to values such as family, spirituality, and career instead of using verbal processes that could lead to choices based on avoidance or social/cultural compliance (Hayes, 1984; Hayes et al., 2006).

ACT treatment involves the initial demonstration that an individual's previous attempts at improving symptoms of distress have not been successful because of the failure of the system within which he/she is working. The next treatment phase involves focusing on the futility of trying to control inner thoughts and emotions. ACT suggests that the problem isn't the thoughts, feelings, or emotions but rather the attempt to avoid, control, or eliminate these experiences (Hayes et al., 2013).

Dialectical Behavior Therapy

DBT was originally developed for the treatment of borderline personality disorder but has since been successfully used with a variety of symptoms including symptoms caused by trauma or stress (Cukor et al., 2009; Haghayegh et al., 2017). There are three foundations of DBT. Behaviorism as a foundation aims to replace negative or maladaptive behaviors with more skillful behaviors. Zen principles as another foundation of DBT inform the skills curriculum and contribute to acceptance instead of avoidance. With this foundation, awareness is informed by more than individual emotion and fact and is influenced by core mindfulness skills. Similar to ACT and MBCT, these mindfulness skills adopt an accepting and non-judgmental attitude toward thoughts, feelings, and emotions. The final foundation of DBT is dialectics, which contributes toward a worldview and a balance between acceptance and change.

The structure of DBT treatment includes individual therapy, skills training (mindfulness, distress tolerance, emotion regulation, and interpersonal effectiveness), consultation with a therapist, and telephone coaching.

The philosophical and theoretical underpinnings of both ACT and DBT are outside of the scope of this book but if you are interested in a more structured intervention for dealing with the traumatic and stressful experiences you are exposed to in nursing or if symptoms of stress are interfering with your ability to function at work or in your personal life, you may want to explore the availability of these treatments. MBCT is also considered a "third-generation" therapy, and you were provided with instructions on practicing a few of the mindfulness practices used in that therapy earlier in this chapter. However, if you would like to explore the benefits of MBCT and whether MBCT could be beneficial to your work as a nurse, there is a structured eight-week program that is delivered in a group setting.

Mindfulness Practice while Working

As discussed previously, it will probably be difficult for you to practice sitting meditation for 10–20 min while you are working. That doesn't mean that mindfulness during work hours isn't important. If you work in a hospital setting with high acuity patients such as the emergency department or the ICU, sometimes being on autopilot is prioritized to make it through a crisis. However, choose the moments when mindfulness can be folded into practice as a method to diffuse strong emotions or ruminative thoughts that are consuming your mind and making it impossible to be present for your patients. If you are currently practicing nursing, think of the number of times you have tossed and turned while trying to sleep at night. Why does that happen? The stories presented in Chapter 3 in addition to your own narratives are powerful examples of the relationship we have with thoughts and emotions.

In addition to the 3-min breathing exercise discussed earlier in this chapter, there are other mindfulness practices that you could try incorporating into your work day.

- *Mindful handwashing*—as a nurse during any given day, you will wash your hands hundreds of times. At a minimum, you are washing your hands any time you enter or exit a patient's room. Instead of being on automatic pilot, be mindful of the temperature of the water on your skin, the smell of the soap, the texture and feel of the soap on your hands, any changes in soap color based on the lighting in the room, and after rinsing the soap off your hands, the way the paper towel feels as you are drying your hands off. This is a 30-s exercise that will help bring awareness to the present moment and, if done multiple times during your shift, can create a cumulative effect, impacting your ability to connect with patients, family members, and coworkers.
- *Mindful eating*—as a nurse, how many times have you eaten so fast during a shift that you can't describe what your food tasted like? I've often heard nurses talk about having to practice eating slowly when they are away from work and having family meals. It's understood that there may be shifts where you don't have time to eat; however, when you are able to take a lunch break, eating mindfully is another mindfulness practice that can be done in the work setting. How does your food look, smell, taste, and feel while you are eating? Where did your food come from (is it organic, where was it grown, is it processed)? Is the food you are eating healthy? Why do you feel like eating (hunger, emotions)? In addition to being a mindfulness practice that you have time for at work, there are also benefits such as learning how to enjoy eating food, learning to only eat when you're hungry, and understanding how emotion effects what you ingest and how food may affect your energy level and mood throughout the day.

■ *Mindful walking*—since the use of FitBits and Apple watches is so common, it's easy to keep up with the number of steps or miles that you've walked during any given time period. Nurses walk a lot! When you are walking to the cafeteria for a dinner break or walking to the pharmacy, laboratory, X-ray, etc. think about walking mindfully. Notice your breath and any changes in your rate of breathing, the floor, and how solid the ground feels beneath your feet; feel the contact of your foot on the ground, which part of your foot touches the ground first; Do you notice any sounds or smells? and if you get distracted with thought, redirect your attention in a non-judgmental way to your breath and the task of walking.

In conclusion, this chapter discusses mindfulness as a resilience intervention that can be used and practiced by nurses to help prevent symptoms of stress, trauma, anxiety, depression, and burnout syndrome, which can be caused by working in the acute care setting. Examples are provided for practicing mindfulness at home and shorter practices that can be done at work. These practices are based on the third-generation psychotherapies, specifically ACT and DBT. There is no effectiveness data on the use of mindfulness interventions for the mitigation of psychological distress; however, pilot results have shown promise and nurses have expressed great satisfaction with engaging in personal mindfulness practices. Future research in this area is needed.

References

American Nurses Association. (2017). Exploring moral resilience toward a culture of ethical practice: A call to action report. Retrieved from: www.nursingworld.org/~4907b6/globalassets/ docs/ana/ana-call-to-action--exploring-moral-resilience-final.pdf.

Bernstein, A., Hadash, Y., Lichtash, Y., Tanay, G., Shepherd, K. & Fresco, D. (2015). Decentering and related constructs: A critical review and metacognitive processes model. *Perspectives on Psychological Science*, 10, 599–617.

Burton, A., Burgess, C., Dean, S., Koutsopoulou, G. & Hugh-Jones, S. (2017). How effective are mindfulness-based interventions for reducing stress among healthcare professionals? A systematic review and meta-analysis. *Stress and Health*, 33, 3–13.

Carlson, L.E., Beattie, T.L., Giese-Davis, J., Faris, P., Tamagawa, R., Fick, L.J., ... & Speca, M. (2015). Mindfulness-based cancer recovery and supportive-expressive therapy maintain telomere length relative to controls in distressed breast cancer survivors. *Cancer*, 121, 476–484.

Cukor, J., Spitalnick, J., Difede, J., Rizzo, A. & Rothbaum, B. (2009). Emerging treatments for PTSD. *Clinical Psychology Review*, 29, 715–726.

Dimidjian, S. & Goodman, S.H. (2014). Preferences and attitudes toward approaches to depression relapse/recurrence prevention among pregnant women. *Behavior Research and Therapy*, 54, 7–11.

Foureur, M., Besley, K., Burton, G., Yu, N. & Crisp, J. (2013). Enhancing the resilience of nurses and midwives: Pilot of mindfulness based program for increased health, sense of coherence and decreased depression, anxiety and stress. *Contemporary Nurse*, 45, 114–125.

Garland, E.L., Froeliger, B. & Howard, M.O. (2015). Neurophysiological evidence for remediation of reward processing deficits in chronic pain and opioid misuse following treatment with mindfulness-oriented recovery enhancement: Exploratory ERP findings from a pilot RCT. *Journal of Behavioral Medicine*, 38, 327–336.

Haghayegh, S., Neshatdoost, H., Adibi, P. & Shafii, F. (2017). Efficacy of dialectical behavior therapy on stress, resilience and coping strategies in irritable bowel syndrome patients. *Research in Medical Sciences*, 19, 1–7.

Hayes, S. (1984). Making sense of spirituality. *Behaviorism*, 12, 99–110.

Hayes, S. (2004). Acceptance and commitment therapy, relational frame theory, and the third wave of behavioral and cognitive therapies. *Behavior Therapy*, 35, 639–665.

Hayes, S., Luoma, J., Bond, F., Masuda, A. & Lillis, J. (2006). Acceptance and commitment therapy: Model, processes and outcomes. *Behaviour Research and Therapy*, 44, 1–25.

Hayes, S., Levin, M., Plumb-Vilardaga, J., Villatte, J. & Pistorello, J. (2013). Acceptance and commitment therapy and contextual behavioral science: Examining the progress of a distinctive model of behavioral and cognitive therapy. *Behavioral Therapy*, 44, 180–198.

Kabat-Zinn, J. (2013). *Full Catastrophe Living*. New York: Random House.

Mealer, M., Conrad, D., Evans, J., Jooste, K., Solyntjes, J., Rothbaum, B. & Moss, M. (2014). Feasibility and acceptability of a resilience training program for intensive care unit nurses. *American Journal of Critical Care*, 23, 97–105.

Mealer, M., Hodapp, R., Conrad, D., Dimidjian, S., Rothbaum, B. & Moss, M. (2017). Designing a resilience program for critical care nurses. *AACN Advanced Critical Care*, 28, 359–365.

Nhat-Hanh, T. (2015). *The Heart of the Buddha's Teaching*. New York: Penguin Random House.

Teasdale, J.D., Segal, Z.V. & Williams, J.M. (1995). How does cognitive therapy prevent depressive relapse in recurrent major depressive disorder: A systematic review and meta-analysis. *Clinical Psychology Review*, 33, 25–39.

Chapter 5

Writing for Wellness

Expressive writing was developed in the 1980s and is founded on the principle that the suppression of previous traumatic events or unresolved stressful events inhibits the ability to cope with current stressful events and/or adversity. Theoretically, if you are able to construct a trauma narrative, the written emotional disclosure allows you to reflect on the negative experience and reconstruct meaning associated with the experience, which allows processing and a newfound relationship with the experience. The earliest studies on expressive writing involved college students who wrote about their most traumatic experience for 15–20 min on 3–5 consecutive days. Expressive writing was associated with improved grades, fewer visits to the infirmary, and better adjustment to college. Since then, over 200 similarly structured randomized trials have been conducted addressing common illnesses, or common stressors such as workplace issues and trauma exposure. These randomized trials and several subsequent meta-analyses have demonstrated that writing generally improves psychological health.

There have been several variations of writing techniques with slightly different underlying philosophies and applications since expressive writing for emotional healing was developed.

One such technique is written exposure therapy (WET), which is a form of written disclosure.

The WET protocol consists of five weekly 30-min writing sessions and is meant to reduce arousal and negative affect among individuals meeting diagnostic criteria for posttraumatic stress disorder (PTSD). It is theorized that confronting a traumatic memory through writing, instead of avoiding the traumatic memory, can provide emotional processing and fear extinction related to the event. What is so encouraging about WET is that it is a brief intervention. Clinical practice guidelines for the management of PTSD involve time-intensive psychotherapies that have a primary component of cognitive restructuring, prolonged exposure, and Cognitive Processing Therapy (CPT). As we learned in previous chapters, nurses have a high prevalence of PTSD and other psychological symptoms as a result of traumatic work experiences.

The idea of a short writing intervention to mitigate stress and the effects of trauma in nursing is encouraging for several reasons including the time commitment required by a nurse, the independence of the intervention (writing can be done just about anywhere and with minimal resources), and the flexibility of initiation since others' schedules are not impacted (no requirement for a therapist). In addition, the feasibility of nurses engaging in traditional psychotherapies is concerning. Not only are the psychotherapies time intensive, but there is also the difficulty of uncertain scheduling patterns and long shift work in nursing, particularly in the acute care setting.

Fortunately, there has been some promising research suggesting that WET may be equally effective for the treatment of PTSD symptoms when compared to the more traditional CPT. A randomized, controlled trial was conducted by Sloan and colleagues (2018) and randomized individuals to either WET or CPT. Subjects were included in the study if they met diagnostic criteria for PTSD and were on stable medication therapy.

Of the 126 participants (63 randomized to each intervention arm), there was no difference in improvements between the two groups, and the WET group had fewer dropouts than the CPT group.

Writing to Improve Resilience in Nursing

To date, we have conducted two studies using a writing therapy intervention, and the results have been promising.

Study One: A Multimodal Resilience Training Program for Intensive Care Unit Nurses

The multimodal resilience intervention involved four components: aerobic exercise, event-triggered cognitive behavioral therapy sessions, mindfulness-based interventions, and expressive writing/WET (described in detail in Chapter 3).

The writing intervention differed from the traditional WET or expressive writing protocols and, instead, combined the two protocols to include 12 weekly writing sessions that prompted participants to write about both work-related trauma and personal trauma or emotional upheavals. The writing prompts were delivered to participants by email each week, each session lasted 20–30 min, and nurses entered their writing session directly into an electronic database. To ensure anonymity and to limit hesitancy by the nurse participants to write about these potentially sensitive topics, the study team and writing experts were blinded to the identity of the writer in the database. However, for safety reasons, there was an unblinded honest broker who held the key to the writing session and the nurse participant. If the writing experts were concerned about a nurse participant's writing content and believed there was a need to involve emergency mental health services, the blind could be broken to provide support.

It is important to note that this was not needed during the study (Mealer et al., 2014).

The writing experts used motivational interviewing and cognitive restructuring to respond to each writing session. They also provided feedback on each session and suggested areas to expand upon during a subsequent writing session.

It is important to note that this study was a pilot study that was aimed at determining whether a multimodal resilience intervention would be feasible and acceptable to an intensive care unit (ICU) nursing population. It was encouraging to note that the nurse participants completed 100% of their writing sessions as designed in the protocol. Additionally, based on a satisfaction survey, there was also a high level of satisfaction with the writing component. The study was not statistically powered to determine whether the intervention was effective, but preliminary pilot results showed a significant reduction in symptoms of PTSD ($p = 0.02$) and a significant increase in individual resilience levels ($p = 0.03$).

Below are a couple of exemplary writing sessions from this study. These are the words of the nurse participant(s); however, names will be changed for privacy purposes. Chapter 3 discussed exemplars, not to exploit the suffering that our nurses are feeling both professionally and personally, but rather as a lens to view a caring profession such as nursing. If you are reading this book as a new graduate nurse or someone who has been a nurse for many years, you are not alone. These thoughts and emotions are common, but unfortunately, there is still stigma surrounding mental health issues and fear around being viewed as "weak" or that you are just not cut out for the nursing profession.

Exemplar #1

"I cried during Mary's family meeting. I didn't bawl or draw attention away from John (her husband), but I cried. I couldn't hold it in. I felt like I should be able to hold it together better.

I felt embarrassed. Did the physicians think I am some uncontrolled overly-empathetic nurse? Were they wondering why I can't get a grip. Don't I do this every day? But I also feel like what is happening to Mary and John is incredibly sad, and maybe they deserve to have that sadness validated by someone who is removed. Maybe.

Maybe I was crying for myself. I pictured my husband Steve being sat down by these people, these doctors I know so well. I pictured them presenting him with the options, the prognosis. I pictured him taking in that information, but also feeling in his heart that there has to be something more we can do, that it isn't time to give up yet.

"As a nurse, does this seem purposeless to you?"

"John, I find a lot of purpose in caring for your wife." And if it were my husband in that bed, we'd be pushing on. If there is even an iota of a chance that she will survive, doesn't she deserve it? She is 26 and newlywed, she has her entire life to live. And everything to live for. We are back in the room now. I told him it is the doctors' responsibility that they feel the weight of needing to tell you how grim the situation is. But in the end, you need to make your decisions based on what is right for you and Mary, regardless of how you perceive the staff to feel about it all. What I didn't say is, you are the one who is going to have to live with it.

I'm not sure if I handled it right. I'm not sure if I should just cry when I feel like the situation is sad enough to merit tears. Is that validating or is it self-serving? Either way, I dreamt the night before I had to return to work. I was thinking of Mary all weekend and wondering if she would be alive when I got back. The weird thing is, I've been back for 2 days and haven't gone over to see her. I'll wear her prayer bracelet, but I can't make myself go over to see her.

So the night before I went back in, I dreamt that I was in a field. Other things had just finished happening—a festival or something. Everyone was walking away. But two people were walking toward me. They were the two hepatologists working with Mary. I recognized them immediately and I knew why they were coming over to me. She was dead.

When they approached me I started crying, just like I had in the meeting. The lead hepatologist didn't say a word, he just laughed at me. He laughed at me and then said, "Why are YOU crying?" I didn't respond because I was too choked up, but I thought, Why doesn't he just say it? Why doesn't he just come out with it and tell me she is dead and then leave me alone to grieve?

But they didn't tell me. They left and I knew she was dead and I came into work the next morning and she was alive."

Exemplar #2

"The most significant emotional experience that I have faced in the last 6 weeks actually happened last week while I was caring for a patient. I had gotten to work and an off service patient was recently admitted. He was a bariatric patient who came from an LTAC who was developmentally delayed and intubated. His wife was also developmentally delayed, but highly functional. This patient was admitted for sepsis and was having low blood pressure.

As I was getting report from the day nurse we noticed that he was more unstable than he had been on day shift. His blood pressure was dropping and his heart rate was very fast and irregular. I called the docs to let them know and suggested that they come by and see him. They came up within 30 min to see this patient and decided to do a few procedures on him early in the night. After about 2 h of getting this patient a central line, an arterial line, and changing his drips the patient was more stable. The orders were to titrate down off LEVOPHED and to start vasopressin and titrate up the phenylephrine as needed for a goal BP.

He had a PICC (peripherally inserted central catheter) line that they thought was infected and wanted it taken out and cultured now that the new central line was placed.

The LEVOPHED was running through this line and so my thought process was to discontinue it once the LEVOPHED had been turned off and he was converted over to phenyleph-rine and vasopressin. At about 02:00 the patient's LEVOPHED was on a very low dose, and there was room to go up on his phenylephrine. I let the bag run dry and was hoping that he wasn't ultra-sensitive to the small dose and that the phenylephrine would be fine to use instead.

During that time the patient's blood pressure tanked— almost to the point he didn't have one. Knowing this patient was super sick and would be hard to resuscitate, I panicked. I had to emergently grab my charge nurse and ask her to get another bag of LEVOPHED for me. Usually we don't have them pre-mixed in our Pyxis, but we recently started stocking them (thank GOD!). I had allowed my whole bag to run dry and the tubing had air in it. We had to prime a whole new primary tubing set and then restart it as quickly as possible. This patient literally had like no blood pressure during this entire event. I thought my heart had stopped.

It felt like it lasted an eternity but in reality it was prob-ably less than 5 min. The patient was fine, his blood pressure recovered and the docs didn't seem too worried about it. I was though. I thought about it for the rest of my shift and it both-ered me for days. My adrenaline was pumping and I think my heart rate was >115 for the rest of the night. I was so angry at myself for not anticipating the worst, as I usually do. I felt it was careless for me to let the bag run dry and not even have a back-up "just in case." Had there not been LEVOPHED already mixed in the Pyxis the outcome could have been much worse.

I'm frustrated that I set my pump to allow the bag to run dry instead of alarming when I had some time left to reevalu-ate the situation. I felt annoyed that he and his wife were both needy on top of all of the problems I was facing with his drips. I felt stupid in front of my charge nurse that I freaked out and made her stress out over finding/mixing a new bag for me as this patient's BP tanked.

I talked about it later with my charge nurse and she told me that I was too amped up about it and that I needed to just let it go. I couldn't though. I found myself talking about it with my fiancé, who is also a nurse before I went to bed, and again when I woke up. I talked to my roommate who is a nurse in the SICU about it, and also to a few of my close co-workers. I thought talking about it and admitting my mistake would make me feel better about it, but it didn't. It helped me put the situation in perspective—being that the patient survived it wasn't that big of a deal in the end, but it didn't make me feel better.

I still worry that my charge nurse thinks I'm an idiot. I have recently taken on more leadership roles on my unit, and I feel like the nurses I was working with now look at me as someone who "lost her cool" during a stressful situation—which I guess I did, I just don't want to be viewed that way. I also am very assertive especially when I'm stressed and I feel like I may have been too demanding that night.

Even though the situation is technically resolved, I still don't feel at ease about it. I feel frustrated with myself. I'm trying to look at this experience in a positive light though. My co-workers and I have joked about it, and I know that I gain their trust in the number of stressful situations that I excel at that definitely outweigh the bad ones. Overall I feel okay about it now, just frustrated that I was hadn't anticipated it."

Study Two: WET for ICU Nurses

We recently conducted a feasibility study of a WET intervention to improve resilience and reduce symptoms of distress in critical care nurses. The WET intervention included five-weekly writing sessions. Each weekly period included having nurse study participants complete a 30-min writing assignment. The nurses were asked to write about a traumatic work experience that they considered to be the most significant event in their career and one that is still causing a level of distress.

During the first session, participants were provided with burnout syndrome (BOS) and PTSD psychoeducation, including the common triggers of BOS and PTSD in the ICU environment, common symptoms associated with both BOS and PTSD, and how avoiding or attempting to avoid reminders of the traumatic events experienced in the ICU can exacerbate symptoms of PTSD. The nurses were also provided with the WET treatment rationale, which emphasized confronting traumatic memories and reminders of the traumatic memories through writing. The information provided during the psychoeducation, and study rationale was also provided in writing so that the nurses could refer back to the information at a later date, if needed.

Next, the study team gave the nurses general instructions about the writing sessions that would follow, such as not worrying about spelling or grammar and trying to write uninterrupted during the session time.

After the first writing session, the remaining session (sessions 2–5) prompts were delivered by email each week. Each writing session was meant to build off the original session related to a significant traumatic experience at work that was still causing a level of distress. The remaining sessions may have involved completing the narrative that was not finished during the first writing session, the emotions and/or feelings that the nurse was experiencing during the event, or whether there are personal regrets related to the event, and how the event made the nurse feel about plans to stay in the nursing profession.

Each writing session was directly entered into an electronic database by the nurse participant. The electronic database was managed by an honest broker so that the participant was anonymous to the study team. After each writing assignment was complete, a certified expressive writing professional read the narrative and provided confidential feedback to each participant with an individualized constructive comment, which was meant to improve cognitive flexibility and reframing. When necessary, participants were encouraged to expand on their subsequent writing session in response to the feedback.

Pre- and post-measures of depression, anxiety, BOS, PTSD, and resilience were administered. A satisfaction survey was also completed after the five-week intervention. One hundred percent of the nurses completed their writing sessions. There were significant improvements in subject resilience scores (74 ± 10.7; 85 ± 10.9, $p = 0.03$). The other measures did not show significant changes; however, the results were trending in a positive direction. There were four central domains that were identified as causing trauma in the workplace including patient death, abuse by a patient, peer relationships, and understaffing. We found that the WET writing intervention was feasible for critical care nurses and that writing about traumatic work experiences has the potential to decrease symptoms of distress and improve resilience by developing a trauma narrative guided by reflection and reconstruction of the event.

Exemplars from this study's writing sessions are provided in Chapter 2.

Developing Your Own Writing Practice

The remaining pages of this chapter will discuss developing your own writing practice for wellness. Table 5.1 provides examples of work-related writing prompts that you can use to get started. If you don't see a topic that you would like to write about, you can come up with your own writing prompt. Write about a work situation, a patient, or an interaction with a coworker. Anything that is connected to your work as a nurse. Take 20–30 min to write without interruption.

Table 5.1 Work-Related Writing Prompts

1. Write about a moment of pain that you experienced on the job.
2. Write about a moment when you felt you would be overcome with emotion, but you could not let it show.
3. Write about a time at work that enters your mind more than you would like.
4. Write about a situation at work that occupies your thinking when you are not at work.
5. Write about something that happened at work that you often dream about.
6. Write about something someone said at work that you can't seem to get out of your mind.
7. Write about a situation at work that conflicted with your personal values.
8. Write about your most traumatic experience at work.
9. Write about what drew you to do the kind of work you do.
10. Write about a patient that you could not save.
11. Write about something at work that you wish you could do over.
12. Write about a time you overcame your fear at work.
13. Write about the moment when you dreaded to report for work.
14. Write about a time at work when you were unable to do what needed to be done.
15. Write about how something you do outside of work has helped you perform better at work.
16. Write about someone at work who exhibits resilience.
17. Write about what you believe is true and valuable about what you bring to your work.
18. Write about how the way you think allows you to do your job?
19. Write about what you are most thankful for at work.
20. Write about something at work that you find extremely funny.
21. Write about hope or despair.
22. Write about a time that you were at your clinical best.
23. Write about an experience of joy at work.
24. Write the story of a time when you were moved by the suffering of another.
25. Write about an interaction with a colleague, either positive or difficult.
26. Write about a mentor who has influenced your work.

(Continued)

Table 5.1 (*Continued*)   Work-Related Writing Prompts

27. Write about a patient that you have not forgotten and what it is that keeps them so alive in your memory. Write about a memorable patient encounter.
28. Write about the meaning of your work in your life.
29. Write about when you experienced someone's undivided attention.
30. Write about a time when you felt you truly "became yourself"/ were true to yourself, through your work.
31. Write about a time of "bearing witness."
32. Write about a time when you were an attentive listener.
33. Write about how you wish to be thought of at work by your patients, your supervisor, or by your colleagues.
34. Write about how you explain what you do at work to your family or friends.
35. Write about what gives you strength to continue doing your work.
36. Write about what would help you do your job better.

Expressive writing to overcome trauma, improve health, and build resilience: In addition to nursing work-related prompts that can be used as a writing tool to cope with work-related trauma and stress, an intervention developed by James Pennebaker and John Evans (2014) guides you through a four-day writing protocol as follows (Table 5.2):

Table 5.2 Expressive Writing about Trauma or Emotional Upheaval

Day One Writing Instructions
Remember that this is the first of 4 days of writing. In today's writing, your goal is to write about your deepest thoughts and feelings about the trauma or emotional upheaval that has been influencing your life the most. In your writing, really let go and explore this event and how it has affected you. Today, it may be beneficial to simply write about the event itself, how you felt when it was occurring, and how you feel now.
As you write about this upheaval, you might begin to tie it to other parts of your life. For example, how is it related to your childhood and your relationships with your parents and close family? How is the event connected to those people you have most loved, feared, or been angry with? How is this upheaval related to your current life—your friends and family, your work, and your place in life? And above all, how is this event related to who you have been in the past, who you would like to be in the future, and who you are now? In today's writing, it is particularly important that you really let go and examine your deepest emotions and thoughts surrounding this upheaval in your life. Remember to write continuously for the entire 20 min. And never forget that this writing is for you and you alone. At the conclusion of your 20 min of writing, read the section "Post-Writing Thoughts" and complete the post-writing questionnaire.

Thoughts Following the Day One Writing Session
Congratulations! You have completed the first day of writing. After each writing exercise, it can be helpful to make objective assessments about how the writing felt. In this way, you can go back and determine which writing methods are most effective for you. For this and for all future writing exercises, respond to each of the five following questions either at the end of your writing or in a separate place. Put a number between 0 and 10 by each question.

0	1	2	3	4	5	6	7	8	9	10
Not at all					Somewhat					A great deal

(Continued)

Table 5.2 (*Continued*)   Expressive Writing about Trauma or Emotional Upheaval

A. ____To what degree did you express your deepest thoughts and feelings? B. ____To what degree do you currently feel sad or upset? C. ____To what degree do you currently feel happy? D. ____To what degree was today's writing valuable and meaningful for you? E. Briefly describe how your writing went today so you may refer to this later.
For many people, the first day of writing is the most difficult. This kind of writing can bring up emotions and thoughts that you may not have known that you had. It may also have flowed much more easily than you expected—especially if you wrote about something that you have been keeping to yourself for a long time. If you don't want anyone to see your writing, keep the pages in a secure place or destroy them. If keeping them is not a problem, you can go back and analyze the pages at the end of the 4 days of writing. Now take some time for yourself. Until tomorrow.
Day Two Writing Instructions
Today is the second day of the four-day process. In your last writing session, you were asked to explore your thoughts and feelings about a trauma or emotional upheaval that has affected you deeply. In today's writing, your task is to really examine your very deepest emotions and thoughts. You can write about the same trauma or upheaval as you did yesterday or a completely different one. The writing instructions today are similar to those of your last writing session. Today, try to link the trauma to other parts of your life. Remember that a trauma or emotional upheaval can often influence every aspect of your life—your relationships with friends and family, how you and others view you, your work, and even how you think about your part. In today's writing, begin thinking about how this upheaval is affecting your life in general. You might also write about how you may be responsible for some of the effects of the trauma. As before, write continuously for the entire 20 min and open up your deepest thoughts and feelings. At the conclusion of your writing, complete the post-writing questionnaire.

(*Continued*)

Table 5.2 (*Continued*)   Expressive Writing about Trauma or Emotional Upheaval

Thoughts Following the Day Two Writing Session

You have completed the second of the four-day writing exercise. Before setting aside your writing for the day, please complete the following questionnaire. Put a number between 0 and 10 by each question.

0	1	2	3	4	5	6	7	8	9	10
Not at all					Somewhat					A great deal

A. ____To what degree did you express your deepest thoughts and feelings?

B. ____To what degree do you currently feel sad or upset?

C. ____To what degree do you currently feel happy?

D. ____To what degree was today's writing valuable and meaningful for you?

E. Briefly describe how your writing went today so you may refer to this later.

You now have 2 days of writing to compare. Look at the numbers on the questionnaire from the first day and from today's writing. How did today compare with your first day? Did you notice that your topic was shifting? How about the way you were writing? Between now and your next writing, think about what you have written. Are you starting to see things in a different light? How is writing affecting your emotions?

Now give yourself a little time to step back from your writing. Until tomorrow.

Day Three Writing Instructions

You have made it through 2 days of writing. After today, you will have only one more day of writing. Tomorrow, then, you need to wrap up your story. Today, however, continue to explore your deepest thoughts and emotions about the topics you have been tackling so far.

On the surface, today's writing assignment is very similar to the earlier assignments. In your writing, you can focus on the same topics you have been examining or you can shift your focus to either another trauma or to some other feature of the same trauma. Your primary goal, however, is to focus on your emotions and thoughts about those events that are affecting your life the most right now.

(*Continued*)

Table 5.2 (*Continued*)   Expressive Writing about Trauma or Emotional Upheaval

It is important that you don't repeat what you have already written in your past exercises. Writing about the same general topic is fine, but you also need to explore it from different perspectives and in different ways. As you write about this emotional upheaval, what are you feeling and thinking? How has this event shaped your life and who you are?

In today's writing, allow yourself to explore those deep issues about which you may be particularly vulnerable. As always, write continuously for the entire 20 min.

Thoughts Following the Day Three Writing Session

0	1	2	3	4	5	6	7	8	9	10
Not at all					Somewhat					A great deal

A. ____To what degree did you express your deepest thoughts and feelings?

B. ____To what degree do you currently feel sad or upset?

C. ____To what degree do you currently feel happy?

D. ____To what degree was today's writing valuable and meaningful for you?

E. Briefly describe how your writing went today so you may refer to this later.

In most studies, the third day of writing is highly significant. People often arrive at critical issues they have been avoiding. Whereas the first two writing sessions can be like putting toes in the water to see if it's too cold, by the third day, some people are ready to jump completely in. A second group of people open up most on the first day. By the third day of writing, this second group sometimes is beginning to run out of steam. Both patterns are associated with improved health.

As with your last writing exercise, try to compare what you have written across the three sessions. What issues are surfacing as most important for you? Have you been surprised by any of your feelings while you were writing? Has the writing provoked any thoughts during the periods that you have been away from it?

(Continued)

Table 5.2 (*Continued*)   Expressive Writing about Trauma or Emotional Upheaval

Remember that tomorrow is the final day of the four-day writing exercise. The instructions for your last assignment will be much like today's. Since it will be the final day, however, think about how you will tie things up. Now pamper yourself a bit. Until tomorrow.
Day Four Writing Instructions
This is the final day of the four-day writing exercise. As with the previous days' writings, explore your deepest emotions and thoughts about those upheavals and issues in your life that are most important and troublesome for you. Stand back and think about the events, issues, thoughts, and feelings that you have disclosed.
In your writing, try to tie up anything that you haven't yet confronted. What are your emotions and thoughts at this point? What things have you learned, lost, and gained as a result of this upheaval in your lie? How will these past events guide your thoughts and actions in the future? Really let go in your writing and be honest with yourself about this upheaval. Do you best to wrap up the entire experience into a meaningful story that you can take with you into the future.
Thoughts Following the Final Writing Session
You have completed the last day of writing. Please complete the following questionnaire using a number between 0 and 10 by each question.

0	1	2	3	4	5	6	7	8	9	10
Not at all					Somewhat					A great deal

A. ____To what degree did you express your deepest thoughts and feelings?

B. ____To what degree do you currently feel sad or upset?

C. ____To what degree do you currently feel happy?

D. ____To what degree was today's writing valuable and meaningful for you?

E. Briefly describe how your writing went today so you may refer to this later.

(*Continued*)

Table 5.2 (*Continued*) Expressive Writing about Trauma or Emotional Upheaval

Today concludes the basic four-day writing exercise. Most people find the last day of writing the least enjoyable. This is often a sign that you are tired of dealing with this trauma and want to get on with other life tasks. In some ways, it is tempting to go back over the various writing samples, questionnaire responses, and personal observations immediately after the fourth writing day. Indeed, it is important to review your writing. However, it is strongly recommended that you take at least 2 or 3 days off from the writing exercise before you do this.

Source: copyright: Pennebaker, J.W. & Evans, J.F. (2014). Expressive Writing: Words that Heal. Enumclaw, WA: Idyll Arbor.

Writing doesn't resonate with everyone. Give it a try! Developing a personal writing practice can be a healthy skill to nurture for times when the depleting stresses of your work and personal life outweigh positive or nurturing events that recharge our caring personalities.

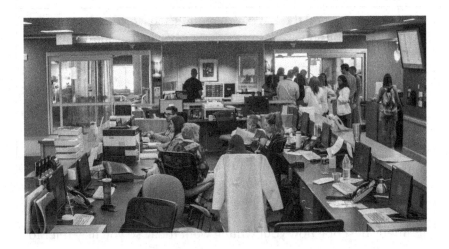

References

Mealer, M., Conrad, D., Evans, J., Jooste, K., Solyntjes, J., Rothbaum, B. & Moss, M. (2014). Feasibility and acceptability of a resilience training program for intensive care unit nurses. *American Journal of Critical Care*, 23, 97–105.

Pennebaker, J.W. & Evans, J.F. (2014). *Expressive Writing: Words that Heal*. Enumclaw, WA: Idyll Arbor.

Index

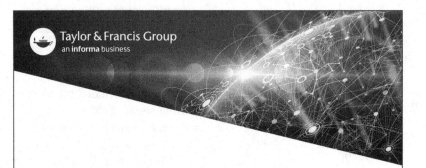